P9-CMK-874

"Mounting evidence indicates that refined carbohydrates and high glycemic index foods are contributing to the escalating epidemics of obesity and type 2 diabetes worldwide. This dietary pattern also appears to increase the risk of heart disease and stroke. The skyrocketing proportion of calories from added sugars and refined carbohydrates in Westernized diets portends a future acceleration of these trends. *The Glucose Revolution* challenges traditional doctrines about optimal nutrition and the role of carbohydrates in health and disease. Brand-Miller and colleagues are to be congratulated for an eminently lucid and important book that explains the science behind the glycemic index and provides tools and strategies for modifying diet to incorporate this knowledge. I strongly recommend the book to both health professionals and the general public who could use this state-of-the-art information to improve health and well-being."

—JOANN E. MANSON, M.D., DR.P.H., Professor of Medicine, Harvard Medical School, and Co-Director of Women's Health, Division of Preventive Medicine, Brigham and Women's Hospital

∎

"Here is at last a book explaining the importance of taking into consideration the glycemic index values of foods for overall health, athletic performance, and in reducing the risk of heart disease and diabetes. The book clearly explains that there are different kinds of carbohydrates that work in different ways and why a universal recommendation to 'increase the carbohydrate content of your diet' is plainly simple and scientifically inaccurate. Everyone should put the glycemic index approach into practice."

—ARTEMIS P. SIMOPOULOS, M.D., senior author of *The Omega Diet* and *The Healing Diet* and President, The Center for Genetics, Nutrition and Health, Washington, D.C., on *The Glucose Revolution*

"*The Glucose Revolution* is nutrition science for the 21st century. Clearly written, it gives the scientific rationale for why all carbohydrates are not created equal. It is a practical guide for both professionals and patients. The food suggestions and recipes are exciting and tasty."

—RICHARD N. PODELL, M.D., M.P.H., Clinical Professor, Department of Family Medicine, UMDNJ-Robert Wood Johnson Medical School, and co-author of *The G-Index Diet: The Missing Link That Makes Permanent Weight Loss Possible*

■

"The glycemic index is a useful tool which may have a broad spectrum of applications, from the maintenance of fuel supply during exercise to the control of blood glucose levels in diabetics. Low glycemic index foods may prove to have beneficial health effects for all of us in the long term. *The Glucose Revolution* is a user-friendly, easy-to-read overview of all that you need to know about the glycemic index. This book represents a balanced account of the importance of the glycemic index based on sound scientific evidence."

—JAMES HILL, PH.D., Director, Center for Human Nutrition, University of Colorado Health Sciences Center

■

"*The New Glucose Revolution* summarizes much of the recent development of dietary glycemic index and load in a highly readable format. The authors are able researchers and respected leaders in the nutrition field. Much that is discussed in this book draws directly from their years of experimental and observational research. The focus on dietary intervention and prevention strategies in everyday eating is an especially laudable feature of this book. I recommend this book most highly as an indispensable source of good nutrition."

—SIMIN LIU, M.D., SC.D., Assistant Professor, Department of Epidemiology, Harvard School of Public Health

■

"As a coach of elite amateur and professional athletes, I know how critical the glycemic index is to sports performance. *The New Glucose Revolution* provides the serious athlete with the basic tools necessary for getting the training table right."

—JOE FRIEL, coach, author, consultant

Other *New Glucose Revolution* Titles

The NEW GLUCOSE Revolution
Low GI Guide to Diabetes

The Quick-Reference Guide to Managing Diabetes Using the Glycemic Index

Dr. Jennie Brand-Miller • Kaye Foster-Powell

Dr. Stephen Colagiuri • Johanna Burani

Da Capo
LIFE LONG

A Member of the Perseus Books Group

Copyright © 2003 by Jennie Brand-Miller, Kaye Foster-Powell, and Stephen Colagiuri
This edition published in somewhat different form in Australia in 2003 under the title The New Glucose Revolution People with Diabetes by Hodder Headline Australia Pty Limited. This edition published by arrangement with Hodder Headline Australia Pty Limited.

The GI logo is a trademark of the University of Sydney in Australia and other countries. A food product carrying this logo is nutritious and has been tested for its GI by an accredited laboratory.

Designed by Pauline Neuwirth, Neuwirth & Associates, Inc.
Set in 10.5 point Fairfield LH by the Perseus Books Group

Cataloging-in-Publication data for this book is available from the Library of Congress.

ISBN: 978-1-56924-335-0

Published by Da Capo Press
A Member of the Perseus Books Group
www.dacapopress.com

Note: The information in this book is true and complete to the best of our knowledge. This book is intended only as an informative guide for those wishing to know more about health issues. In no way is this book intended to replace, countermand, or conflict with the advice given to you by your own physician. The ultimate decision concerning care should be made between you and your doctor. We strongly recommend you follow his or her advice. Information in this book is general and is offered with no guarantees on the part of the authors or Da Capo Press. The authors and publisher disclaim all liability in connection with the use of this book. The names and identifying details of people associated with events described in this book have been changed. Any similarity to actual persons is coincidental.

10 9 8 7 6 5 4 3 2

CONTENTS

PREFACE

*T*HE *NEW GLUCOSE REVOLUTION* is the definitive, all-in-one guide to the glycemic index. Now we have written this pocket guide to show you how the glycemic index (GI) can help you achieve better control of your diabetes. As we explain in *The New Glucose Revolution*, the glycemic index:

- ◗ is a proven guide to the true physiological effects foods—especially carbohydrates—have on blood sugar levels
- ◗ provides an easy and effective way to eat a healthy diet and control fluctuations in blood sugar

This book offers more in-depth information about using the glycemic index to manage diabetes than we had room to include in *The New Glucose Revolution*.

Much new information appears in this book that is not in *The New Glucose Revolution,* including a week's worth of low-GI meal plans, and success stories about diabetics who have made the switch to low-GI foods— and in the process have achieved better control of their blood glucose levels.

This book has been written to be read alongside *The New Glucose Revolution,* so, in the event you haven't already, please consult that book for a more comprehensive discussion of the glycemic index and all its uses.

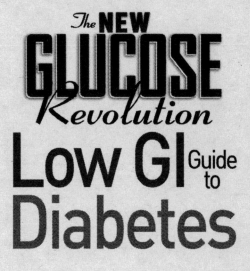

The NEW
GLUCOSE
Revolution
Low GI Guide
to
Diabetes

◀ 1 ▶

WHAT THIS BOOK
CAN DO FOR YOU

*D*ID YOU KNOW that seventeen million people—
6.2 percent of the U.S. population—have diabetes? Yet only about eleven million of those people have
actually been diagnosed with the disease; the remaining
six million don't even know they're sick. Every year,
health professionals diagnose more than one million new
cases of the disease in people ages twenty and older.

In fact, many people don't even know they are suffer-
ing from the sixth leading cause of death in the United
States until they develop one of its life-threatening com-
plications such as blindness, kidney disease, nerve damage, heart disease, or stroke.

THE IMPORTANCE OF A GOOD DIET

The good news? You can control many diabetic symp-
toms by getting regular medical check-ups, enjoying

plenty of exercise and eating a healthy diet. That's how this book can help. Health authorities all over the world stress the importance of high carbohydrate diets for good health and diabetes management. The question now is which type of carbohydrate is best for people with diabetes? Research on the glycemic index (what we call the GI) shows that different carbohydrate foods have dramatically different effects on blood sugar levels.

■

The glycemic index gives you the true story about the carbohydrate–blood sugar connection. For people with diabetes this can mean a new lease on life . . . literally!

■

Understanding the glycemic index has made an enormous difference to the diet and lifestyle of people with diabetes because the findings reveal that:

- many traditionally forbidden foods actually don't cause an unhealthy rise of glucose in the blood as was once believed
- diets containing low-GI foods improve blood sugar control in people with type 1 (insulin-dependent) and type 2 (non-insulin-dependent) diabetes
- using foods low on the glycemic index widens the choices for people with diabetes for healthy and enjoyable eating

WHAT IS THE GLYCEMIC INDEX?

The glycemic index is a ranking of foods based on their immediate effect on blood sugar levels. Carbohydrate foods that break down quickly during digestion have the highest GI values because their blood sugar response is fast and high. Carbohydrate foods that break down slowly, releasing glucose gradually into the bloodstream, have low GI values.

The rate of carbohydrate digestion has important implications for everybody. It's vital that people with diabetes learn about the glycemic index so they can base their food choices on sound scientific evidence. (For more information about the glycemic index, see Chapter 6.)

HOW TO USE THIS BOOK

Many people with diabetes find that, despite doing all they are told, their blood sugar levels remain too high. This book contains the most up-to-date information about carbohydrate and the optimum meal-planning approach for people with diabetes. It explains which types of carbohydrate are best and why—information based on scientific research, clinical trials, and the real experiences of real people. This Pocket Guide:

▶ shows you how to include more of the right type of carbohydrate in your diet
▶ provides practical hints for meal preparation and tips to help you make the glycemic index work for you throughout the day

- gives a week of low-GI menus plus a nutritional analysis for each menu and its glycemic index
- explains how scientists measure the glycemic index
- includes an A to Z listing of 375 foods with their GI values, glycemic load, and carbohydrate and fat counts

◀ 2 ▶

TREAT DIABETES
WITH A LOW-GI DIET

*O*NE OF THE major aims of diabetes therapy is to maintain near normal blood sugar levels. Not long ago, people with diabetes were told to eat complex carbohydrates (starches) because it was believed they were slowly absorbed by the body and therefore caused a smaller rise in blood sugar levels. Simple sugars were restricted because they were thought to be quickly absorbed and their blood sugar response would therefore be fast and high.

These assumptions were wrong! We now know that the concept of simple and complex carbohydrates doesn't tell us how carbohydrate will actually behave in the body. Different carbohydrate-containing foods do have different effects on blood sugar levels, but we can't predict the effect by looking at their sugar or starch content.

WHAT DOES THE GLYCEMIC INDEX MEAN FOR PEOPLE WITH DIABETES?

Since the 1980s, scientists have studied healthy and diabetic blood sugar responses to hundreds of different foods. Test subjects were given real foods and their blood sugar levels were measured at frequent intervals for two to three hours after the meal. To compare foods according to their true physiological effect on blood sugar levels, they came up with the term "glycemic index" (GI). This is simply a ranking of foods from 0 to 100 that tells us whether a food will raise blood sugar levels dramatically, moderately, or just a little.

■

It's time to forget about simple and complex carbohydrate and to think in terms of low GI foods and high GI foods.

■

Research on the glycemic index has turned some widely held beliefs upside down. The surprises:

- Many starchy foods (some types of bread and potato and many types of rice) are digested and absorbed very quickly—not slowly as we had always assumed.
- Moderate amounts of many sugary foods did not produce the dramatic rises in blood sugar that we had thought.

The Pancreas Produces Insulin

THE PANCREAS IS a vital organ near the stomach, and its main job is to produce the hormone insulin. Carbohydrate stimulates the secretion of insulin more than any other component of food. The slow absorption of the carbohydrate in our food means that the pancreas doesn't have to work so hard and needs to produce less insulin. If the pancreas is overstimulated over a long period of time, it may become "exhausted" and type 2 diabetes can develop in genetically susceptible people. Even without diabetes, high insulin levels are undesirable because they increase the risk of heart disease.

Unfortunately, over time, we have begun to eat more "refined" foods and fewer "whole" foods. This new way of eating has brought with it higher blood sugar levels after a meal and higher insulin responses, as well. Though our bodies do need insulin for carbohydrate metabolism, high levels of the hormone have a profound effect on the development of many diseases. In fact, medical experts now believe that high insulin levels are one of the key factors responsible for heart disease and hypertension. Insulin influences the way we metabolize foods, determining whether we burn fat or carbohydrate to meet our energy needs, and ultimately determining whether we store fat in our bodies.

The truth was that many foods containing sugar actually showed intermediate blood sugar responses, often lower than some types of bread, for example. So, you can forget the old distinctions that we used to make between starchy foods and sugary foods or simple versus complex carbohydrate. These distinctions have meaning in a chemistry textbook to explain the chemical *structure* of these foods, but they don't tell the true story of *what the body does with these foods*. It's the glycemic index that tells the true story.

WHY IS THE GLYCEMIC INDEX SO IMPORTANT IN DIABETES MANAGEMENT?

If blood sugar levels are not properly controlled, diabetes can cause damage to the blood vessels in the eyes, kidneys, and nerves. For this reason, heart attacks, strokes, kidney failure, and blindness are more common in people with diabetes. High blood sugar levels can also damage the nerves in the feet, which can cause pain, irritation and loss of sensation in the feet.

High insulin levels can also damage the blood vessels of the heart, legs, and brain. In fact, some researchers think that high insulin levels might cause the muscle in the walls of blood vessels to thicken. This thickening would cause the blood vessels to narrow and slow the flow of blood. A clot could form and stop the blood flow altogether, causing a heart attack or stroke.

■

The optimum diet for people with diabetes contains a wide variety of foods.

■

In general, studies show an excellent correlation between the glycemic index of a food and its insulin response. With low-GI foods, there's a reduced secretion of the hormone insulin over the course of the day. With high-GI foods, the body produces larger amounts of insulin, resulting in higher levels of insulin in the blood.

It makes sense for people with type 2 diabetes to eat foods with low GI values to help control blood sugar levels, and do so with lower levels of insulin. (A low-GI diet improves the body's sensitivity to insulin, so the insulin you do have works better.) This may have the added benefit of reducing the large vessel damage that accounts for many of the problems that diabetes can cause.

We also know that a low-GI diet in conjunction with a low fat intake can help keep your blood vessels healthy by keeping your levels of blood fats down. Studies have shown that people have lower levels of blood fats (such as cholesterol and triglycerides) when they eat lower-GI foods.

THE KEY IS THE RATE OF DIGESTION

Here's how digestion impacts the glycemic index of a food: Carbohydrate foods that break down quickly during digestion have the highest GI values. Conversely, carbohydrates that break down slowly, releasing glucose gradually into the bloodstream, have low GI values. (For most people most of the time, low-GI foods have advantages over high-GI foods.)

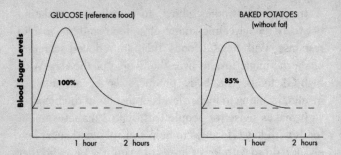

Figure 1. The effect of pure glucose (50 g) and baked potatoes without fat (50 g carbohydrate portion) on blood sugar levels.

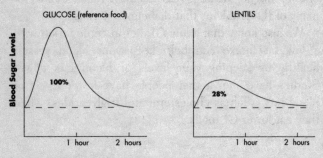

Figure 2. The effect of pure glucose (50 g) and lentils (50 g carbohydrate portion) on blood sugar levels.

The higher the glycemic index, the higher the blood sugar levels after consumption of the food. Rice Krispies (GI value of 82) and baked potatoes (GI value of 85) have very high GI values, meaning their effect on blood sugar levels is almost as high as that of an equal amount of pure glucose (yes, you read it correctly).

Figure 1 shows the blood sugar response to potatoes compared with pure glucose. Foods with a low glycemic index (such as lentils, with an average value of 28) show a flatter blood sugar response when eaten, as shown in

Figure 2. The peak blood sugar level is lower and the return to baseline levels is slower than with a high-GI food.

GI Ranges

Low GI	0–55
Intermediate GI	56–69
High GI	70 or higher

■

The slow digestion and gradual rise and fall in
blood sugar after eating a low-GI food
help control blood sugar levels in people with diabetes.

■

WHAT IS THE OPTIMUM DIET FOR PEOPLE WITH DIABETES?

For over a hundred years, people with diabetes have been given advice on what to eat. Many diets were based more on unproven (although seemingly logical) theories, rather than actual research. In 1915, for example, the *Boston Medical and Surgical Journal* advocated that the best dietary treatment for someone with diabetes was "limitation of all components of the diet." This translated to a very low-calorie diet interspersed with days of fasting. Unfortunately, malnutrition was often the result!

Fortunately, good quality scientific research supports today's dietary recommendations for people with diabetes.

Checklist: The Optimum Diet for People with Diabetes

EATING A HEALTHY diet is easy once you've mastered a few basic concepts. To manage your diabetes properly, you need to eat:

✓ Plenty of whole grain cereals, breads, vegetables, and fruits. A low fat, low-GI diet contains lots of dense, heavy whole grain breads; whole grain cereals such as rice, barley, couscous, cracked wheat; legumes such as kidney beans and lentils; and all types of fruit and vegetables.

✓ Only small amounts of fat, especially saturated fat. Limit cookies, cakes, butter, potato chips, fried fast foods, whole milk dairy products and fatty meats and sausages, which are all high in saturated fat. Polyunsaturated and monounsaturated oils (as found in olives and olive oil, peanuts and peanut oil, canola and fish oils) are healthier types of fats.

✓ A moderate amount of sugar and sugar containing foods. It's okay to include your favorite sweetener or sweet food—small quantities of sugar, honey, syrup, and jam—to make meals more palatable and enjoyable.

✓ Only a moderate quantity of alcohol. Limit your alcohol consumption to two drinks (for men) and one drink (for women) per day, with at least two alcohol-free days a week.

✓ Only a moderate amount of salt and salted foods. Boost flavors by using lemon juice, fresh ground black pepper, garlic, chili, herbs and other seasonings rather than adding salt to your food.

■

A diet that is good for people with diabetes
is a diet that is good for everyone.

■

HOW DOES FOOD
AFFECT OUR BLOOD SUGAR?

Our bodies burn fuel all the time, and the fuel our bodies like best is carbohydrate, which is the only fuel that the brain and red blood cells can use.

When we eat carbohydrate foods, the body breaks them down in the gut into a form of energy that can be absorbed and used by the cells. This process is called digestion. Digestion starts in the mouth when amylase, the digestive enzyme in saliva, is incorporated into the food by chewing. The activity of this enzyme stops in the stomach. Most of the digestion continues only when the carbohydrate reaches the small intestine.

In the small intestine, amylase from pancreatic juice breaks down the large molecules of starch into short chain molecules. These and any disaccharide sugars are then broken into simpler monosaccharides by enzymes in the wall of the intestine. The monosaccharides that result—glucose, fructose, and galactose—are absorbed from the small intestine into the bloodstream.

■

Carbohydrate is the only part of food
that directly affects blood sugar levels.

■

The body responds to the resulting rise in glucose by releasing insulin, which clears the sugar from the blood by moving it into the muscles and cells where it is used for energy. Some glucose stays in the blood to serve the brain and central nervous system.

There are still people who think that because carbohydrate raises blood sugar, people who have diabetes should not eat it at all. This is wrong: Carbohydrate is a necessary part of a healthy diet. For people with diabetes, choosing carbohydrate foods with a low glycemic index flattens out the peaks and valleys in blood sugar and helps achieve more stable blood sugar levels.

- People with type 1 diabetes need to balance the amount and timing of their meals with their dose of insulin and their activity level—rarely an easy task.
- People with type 2 diabetes should distribute their carbohydrate intake throughout the day and may need to consider the timing of their meals in relation to any diabetes medications they take.

■

At least half of our total daily calories should come from carbohydrate.

■

◀ 3 ▶

EIGHT DIABETES MYTHS— DISPELLED

$\mathcal{R}$ESEARCH INTO THE glycemic index shows that some of the popular beliefs about food and diabetes just aren't true. Below, we separate the facts from the fallacies.

MYTH 1:
SUGAR IS THE WORST THING FOR PEOPLE WITH DIABETES.

There is absolute consensus that sugar does not cause diabetes. Sugar and sugary foods in normal portions have no greater effect on blood sugar levels than many starchy foods. Saturated fat is far worse for people with diabetes.

- Type 1 diabetes is an autoimmune health problem triggered by unknown environmental factors, possibly viruses.
- Type 2 diabetes is strongly hereditary and lifestyle factors such as insufficient exercise and excess

weight increase the risk of developing it. Because the dietary treatment of diabetes in the past involved strict avoidance of sugar, many people wrongly believed that sugar was in some way implicated as a cause of the disease.

MYTH 2:
ALL COMPLEX CARBOHYDRATES OR STARCHES ARE SLOWLY DIGESTED IN THE INTESTINE.

Not true. Some starch, such as that in mashed potatoes, is digested quickly, causing a greater change in blood sugar level than many sugar-containing foods.

MYTH 3:
STARCHY FOODS SUCH AS BREAD AND POTATOES ARE FATTENING.

Not true. Bread and pasta are carbohydrate (fuel) foods—the types of foods your body burns most readily. They are the least likely to be stored as body fat.

MYTH 4:
EATING A LOT OF SUGAR CAUSES DIABETES.

Not true. A diet high in fat and quickly digested carbohydrates contributes to obesity, which makes type 2 diabetes more likely to appear in those who are at risk.

MYTH 5:
YOU CAN'T LOSE WEIGHT EATING BETWEEN-MEAL SNACKS.

Not true. The type and total amount of calories consumed and the amount of calories the body uses determine body weight. You can safely include low-fat, high-carbohydrate snacks in a low calorie eating plan.

MYTH 6:
SUGAR IS FATTENING.

Not true. Sugar is just another carbohydrate, and it's almost impossible to turn it into body fat when it's eaten in appropriate amounts.

MYTH 7:
HIGH BLOOD SUGAR IS CAUSED BY EATING TOO MUCH SUGAR.

Not true. A number of factors can cause blood sugar levels to rise. These include the body's response to stress or illness, reduced activity, missed medications, and excess carbohydrate.

MYTH 8:
SUGAR IN THE DIET WILL RESULT IN LOWER INTAKE OF VITAMINS AND MINERALS.

Not true. Studies show that diets containing moderate amounts of refined sugars (10 to 12 percent of calories) are perfectly healthy and that sugar helps make many nutritious foods (oatmeal, for example) more palatable. Diets high in natural sugar from a range of sources, including dairy foods and fruit, often have higher levels of micronutrients such as calcium, riboflavin, and vitamin C.

◀ 4 ▶

WHY WE NEED CARBOHYDRATE

*O*UR BODIES BURN fuel all the time, and the fuel our bodies like best is carbohydrate. Carbohydrate is the *only* fuel the brain and red blood cells can use, and the main source of energy for the muscles during strenuous exercise. Carbohydrate is a vital energy source and you can't afford to leave it out. Carbohydrates, however, were not created equal—you must choose the right kind of carbohydrate for your lifestyle.

WHAT IS CARBOHYDRATE?

Carbohydrate is the starchy part of foods such as rice, bread, potatoes, and pasta. It is also the essential ingredient of sweet foods: The sugars in fruit and honey are carbohydrates, as are the refined sugars in soft drinks and confectionery. Carbohydrate mainly comes from plant foods, such as grains, fruit, vegetables, and legumes (peas and beans). Milk products also contain carbohydrate in the form of milk sugar or lactose. Lactose is the first carbohydrate we encounter as infants, and human milk is higher in lactose than any other mammal milk. It accounts for almost half the energy available to the infant. Some foods contain a large amount of carbohydrate (such as cereals, potatoes, and legumes), while other foods are very dilute sources, such as carrots, broccoli, and salad vegetables. Foods high in carbohydrate include:

- ▶ **grains** including rice, wheat, oats, barley, rye and anything made from them (bread, pasta, noodles, flour, breakfast cereal)
- ▶ **all fruits** such as apples, bananas, grapes, peaches, melons
- ▶ **starchy vegetables** such as potatoes, yams, sweet corn, taro and sweet potato
- ▶ **legumes** including baked beans, lentils, kidney beans, and chickpeas
- ▶ **dairy products** such as milk, yogurt, and ice cream

Sources of Carbohydrate

PERCENTAGE OF CARBOHYDRATE (grams per 3.5 oz of food) in food as eaten:

sugar	100%
cornflakes	85%
tapioca	85%
wheat biscuit	62%
rice	79%
sultanas	75%
flour	73%
water cracker	71%
pasta	70%
barley	61%
oats	61%
bread	47%
split peas	45%
ice cream	22%
banana	21%
sweet potato	17%
sweet corn	16%
grapes	15%
potato	15%
pear	12%
apple	12%
baked beans	11%
orange	8%
peas	8%
plum	6%
milk	5%

5 KEYS TO A HEALTHY DIET

1. Eat carbohydrate-rich foods at every meal and make sure that carbohydrates and vegetables form a large proportion of the meal.
2. Eat carbohydrate-rich foods for snacks, rather than high-fat foods.
3. Include at least the minimum quantity of carbohydrate foods suggested for small eaters (see page 24).
4. Make at least half your carbohydrate choices foods with a low GI value.
5. Do not eat too much fat. High-fat foods are a concentrated source of calories. It takes only a little extra of them to throw your diet out of balance.

■

A healthy diet is high in carbohydrate and low in fat.

■

To improve the quality of our diet most of us need to eat more carbohydrate and less fat.

◀ 5 ▶

ASSESS YOUR
CARBOHYDRATE NEEDS

*Y*OUR CALORIE (AND carbohydrate) requirements depend on your age, gender, activity level, and body size; it's not possible to publish standard figures that will apply to everyone. If you want to assess your own specific calorie requirements and calculate exactly how much carbohydrate you need, we suggest that you consult a dietitian.

Once you have the right amount of carbohydrate in your diet, the next step is to choose the right type of carbohydrate foods—those with low GI values.

•

To improve the quality of our diet most of us need to eat more carbohydrate and less fat.

•

HOW MUCH CARBOHYDRATE DO YOU NEED?

About half of our total calorie intake should come from carbohydrate. A good rule of thumb is to consume 125 grams of carbohydrate for every 1000 calories.

- ● For a low-calorie diet (1200 calories), it means eating about 150 grams of carbohydrate per day.
- ● For a young, active person with higher energy requirements (around 2000 calories), it means eating 250 grams of carbohydrate per day.

We have calculated sample carbohydrate intakes for both small and bigger eaters.

CARBOHYDRATE REQUIREMENTS
FOR SMALL EATERS

You might consider yourself a small eater if you:

- ● are a small-framed female
- ● have a small appetite
- ● do very little physical activity
- ● are trying to lose weight

Even the smallest eater needs these carbohydrate foods every day. This food list supplies 188 grams of carbohydrate, suitable for a 1500-calorie diet.

- ● about four slices of bread (4 oz) or the equivalent (crackers, rolls, English muffins)

plus

- about three small pieces of fruit or the equivalent (fresh, canned, dried)

plus

- 1 cup of high-carbohydrate (starchy) vegetables (corn, legumes, sweet potato)

plus

- at least 1 cup of breakfast cereal or grain (cooked rice or pasta, barley, quinoa, or other grain)

plus

- 2 cups of low fat milk or the equivalent (yogurt, ice cream); this includes milk in your tea and coffee and with your cereal

CARBOHYDRATE REQUIREMENTS FOR BIGGER EATERS

You're a bigger eater if you are:

- an active young female of average frame size
- doing regular physical activity (but not prolonged strenuous exercise)
- an active adult male or teenage boy
- working as a laborer

The following food list provides 313 grams of carbohydrate which is suitable for a 2500-calorie diet.

- about six slices of bread (6 oz) or the equivalent (crackers, rolls, English muffins)

plus

- about three medium sized pieces of fruit or the equivalent (fresh, canned, dried) *plus*

▶ 2 cups of high-carbohydrate vegetables (corn, legumes, sweet potato) and at least 1 cup of raw vegetables

plus

▶ at least 2 cups of cereal or grain food (breakfast cereal or cooked rice, or pasta or other grain)

plus

▶ 2 cups of low-fat milk or the equivalent (yogurt, ice cream); this includes milk in your tea and coffee and with your cereal

The Sugar-Fat Seesaw

DID YOU KNOW that fat and sugar tend to show a reciprocal or seesaw relationship in the diet? Research shows that diets high in fat are low in sugar, and diets low in fat are high in sugar. But studies over the past decade have found that diets high in sugar are no less nutritious than low-sugar diets. This is because restricting sugar is frequently followed by higher fat consumption, and most fatty foods are poor sources of nutrients.

In some cases, high-sugar diets have been found to have higher micronutrient contents. This is because sugar is often used to sweeten some very nutritious foods, such as yogurts, breakfast cereals, and milk.

A low-sugar (and high-fat) diet has more proven disadvantages than a high-sugar (and low-fat) diet.

◀ 6 ▶

SOME BACKGROUND ON THE GLYCEMIC INDEX

WHAT IS THE GLYCEMIC INDEX?

*T*HE GLYCEMIC INDEX of foods is simply a ranking of foods based on their immediate effect on blood sugar levels. To make a fair comparison, all foods are compared with a reference food such as pure glucose and are tested in equivalent carbohydrate amounts. The glycemic index is a scientifically validated tool in the dietary management of diabetes and weight reduction.

Originally, research into the glycemic index of foods was inspired by the desire to identify the best foods for people with diabetes. But scientists are now discovering that the glycemic index has implications for everyone.

Today we know the glycemic index of hundreds of different food items—both generic and name-brand—that have been tested following a standardized testing method. The tables in the back of this book give the glycemic

index of a range of common foods, mainly tested at the
University of Toronto and the University of Sydney.

THE GLYCEMIC INDEX MADE SIMPLE

As we mentioned, carbohydrate foods that break down
quickly during digestion have the highest GI values. The
blood glucose, or sugar, response is fast and high. In
other words the glucose in the bloodstream increases
rapidly. On the other hand, carbohydrates that break
down slowly, releasing glucose gradually into the bloodstream, have low GI values. An analogy might be the
popular fable of the tortoise and the hare. The hare, just
like high-GI foods, speeds away full steam ahead, but
loses the race to the slow but steady tortoise. Similarly,
slow and steady low-GI foods produce a smooth blood
sugar curve without wild fluctuations.

For most people most of the time, the foods with a
low glycemic index have advantages over those with high
GI values. Figure 3 shows the effect of slow and fast carbohydrate on blood sugar levels.

The substance that produces the greatest rise in
blood sugar levels is pure glucose itself. All other foods
have less effect when fed in equal amounts of carbohydrate. The glycemic index of pure glucose is set at 100,
and every other food is ranked on a scale from 0 to 100
according to its actual effect on blood sugar levels.

The glycemic index of a food cannot be predicted
from its composition or the glycemic index of related
foods. To test the glycemic index, you need real people
and real foods. We describe how the glycemic index of a
food is measured in the following section. There is no

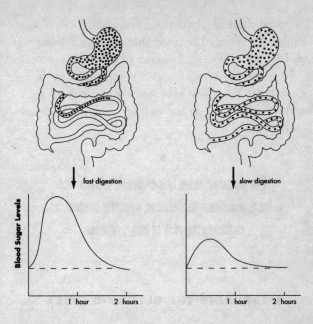

Figure 3. Slow and fast carbohydrate digestion and the consequent levels of sugar in the blood.

easy, inexpensive substitute test. Scientists always follow standardized methods so that results from one group of people can be directly compared with those of another group.

In total, eight to ten people need to be tested, and the glycemic index of the food is the average value of the group. We know this average figure is reproducible and that a different group of volunteers will produce a similar result. Results obtained from diabetics and non-diabetics are comparable.

The most important point to note is that all foods are tested in equivalent carbohydrate amounts. For example,

100 grams of bread (about three and a half slices of sandwich bread) is tested because this contains 50 grams of carbohydrate. Likewise, 2 ounces of jelly beans (containing 50 grams of carbohydrate) is compared with the reference food. We know how much carbohydrate is in a food by consulting food composition tables or the manufacturer's data.

■

**The glycemic index is a clinically proven tool
in its applications to diabetes, appetite control, and
reducing the risk of heart disease.**

■

MEASURING THE GLYCEMIC INDEX

Scientists use just six steps to determine the glycemic index of a food. Simple as this may sound, it's actually quite a time-consuming process. Here's how it works.

1. An amount of food containing 50 grams of carbohydrate is given to a volunteer to eat. For example, to test boiled spaghetti, the volunteer would be given 200 grams of spaghetti, which supplies 50 grams of carbohydrate (we work this out from food composition tables)—50 grams of carbohydrate is equivalent to 3 tablespoons of pure glucose powder.
2. Over the next two hours (or three hours if the volunteer has diabetes), we take a sample of their blood every 15 minutes during the first hour and every 30 minutes thereafter. The blood sugar level

of these blood samples is measured in the laboratory and recorded.

3. The blood sugar level is plotted on a graph and the area under the curve is calculated using a computer program (Figure 4).

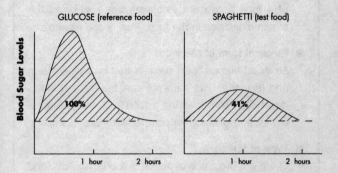

Figure 4. Measuring the glycemic index of a food. The effect of a food on blood sugar levels is calculated using the area under the curve (shaded area). The area under the curve after consumption of the test food is compared with the same area after the reference food (usually 50-g of pure glucose or a 50-g carbohydrate portion of white bread).

4. The volunteer's response to spaghetti (or whatever food is being tested) is compared with his or her blood sugar response to 50 grams of pure glucose (the reference food).

5. The reference food is tested on two or three separate occasions and an average value is calculated. This is done to reduce the effect of day-to-day variation in blood sugar responses.

6. The average glycemic index found in eight to ten people is the glycemic index of that food.

Key Factors that Influence the Glycemic Index

■ **Cooking methods**

Cooking and processing increases the glycemic index of a food because it increases the swelling of the starch molecules in the food. Rice is one example.

■ **Physical form of the food**

An intact fibrous coat, such as that on whole grains and legumes, acts as a physical barrier and slows down digestion, lowering a food's GI value. Beans, barley, and whole grain pumpernickel are examples.

■ **Type of starch**

There are two types of starch in foods, amylose and amylopectin. The more amylose starch a food contains, the lower the glycemic index.

■ **Particle size**

The smaller the particle size, the easier it is for water and enzymes to penetrate. This is why enriched wheat flour (which is a highly processed finely milled flour) has a high GI value, while stone-ground flour, with larger particles, has a lower GI value.

■ **Fiber**

Viscous, soluble fibers, such as those found in rolled oats and apples, slow down digestion and lower a food's glycemic index.

■ **Sugar**

The presence of sugar, as well as the type of sugar, will influence a food's glycemic index. Fruits with a

continued

low glycemic index, such as apples and oranges, are high in fructose. The presence of sugar also will restrict gelatinization (or swelling) of starch that is also present in a food by binding with the water in the food. So some cookies and breakfast cereals that contain sugar may have relatively low GI values.

■ Acidity
Acids in foods slow down stomach emptying, thereby slowing the rate at which the starch can be digested. Vinegar, lemon juice, lime juice, salad dressings, pickled vegetables, and sourdough bread are good examples.

■ Fat
Fat slows down the rate of stomach emptying, thereby slowing the digestion of the starch. For example, potato chips have a lower GI value than boiled potatoes.

◀ 7 ▶

OUR DIETS NEED AN OVERHAUL

$\mathcal{T}$ODAY'S WESTERN DIET is the product of industrialization. It arises in part from widespread use of such inventions as Jethro Tull's seed drill (1701) and high-speed steel roller mills for milling cereals (19th century). Industrialization brought many advances in processing that give many foods longer shelf lives.

The benefits are many: We have plenty of relatively cheap, palatable, and safe foods available, and gone are the days of monotonous fare, gaps in the food supply, and weevil-infested and adulterated food. Also long gone are widespread vitamin deficiencies such as scurvy and pellagra. Today's food manufacturers work hard to bring us irresistible products that meet the demands of both gourmets and health-conscious consumers.

Many of the new foods are still based on our staple cereals—wheat, corn, and oats—but the original grain has been ground down to produce fine flours that yield the best quality breads, cakes, cookies, breakfast cereals, and snack foods.

Cereal chemists and bakers know that the most finely ground flour produces the most palatable and shelf-stable end products. But this striving for excellence in one area has resulted in unforeseen problems in another. Today's staple carbohydrate foods, including some ordinary breads, are quickly digested and absorbed, and the resulting effect on blood sugar levels has created a problem for many of us.

■

Traditional diets all around the world contained slowly digested and absorbed carbohydrate—low-GI foods. In contrast, modern diets with their quickly digested fine white flours are based on high-GI foods.

■

TOO MUCH FAT

The other undesirable aspect of the modern diet is its high fat content. Food manufacturers, bakers and chefs know we love to eat fat. We love its creaminess and texture in the mouth, and we find it easy to consume it in excess. It makes our meat more tender, our vegetables and salads more palatable, and our sweet foods even tastier. We prefer potatoes as French fries or potato chips, to have our fish battered and fried, and our pastas in rich creamy sauces. With a wave of the fat wand, bland high carbohydrate foods such as rice and oats are magically transformed into delicious, calorie-laden foods such as fried rice and sweetened granola. In fact, when you analyze it, much of our diet today is an unwanted but delicious combination of both fat and quickly digested carbohydrate.

WHAT'S WRONG WITH OUR WAY OF EATING?

- ◆ The modern diet is too high in saturated fat and quick-release carbohydrate.
- ◆ The carbohydrate we eat is digested and absorbed too quickly because most modern starchy foods are highly processed and have a high glycemic index.

WHY WE NEED TO EAT
MORE CARBOHYDRATE

For once, health experts agree almost unanimously. The food we eat for breakfast, lunch, and dinner, and for those in-between snacks, should be low in fat and high in carbohydrate. The same diet that helps prevent our becoming overweight also reduces our risk of developing heart disease, diabetes, and many types of cancer. (This same high carbohydrate and low-fat diet also improves athletic performance. For more information on that subject, read our companion guide, *The Glucose Revolution Pocket Guide to Sports Nutrition*.)

But the story doesn't end there. To reduce the fat content of our diet, we need to eat more carbohydrate. In fact, carbohydrate should be the main source of calories in our food—not fat. Carbohydrate and fat have a reciprocal relationship in our diets: If we eat more high-carbohydrate foods, they tend to displace the high-fat foods from our diet.

WHAT IS A BALANCED DIET?

It makes sense to balance our food intake with the rate our bodies use it in order to maintain a steady weight. These days, however, this balance is difficult to achieve, since it's so easy to overeat and under-move. Refined foods, convenience foods, and fast foods usually lack fiber and conceal fat so that, before we feel full, we have overdosed on calories. It is even easier not to exercise. It takes longer to walk somewhere than it does to drive (except perhaps in rush hour). With intake exceeding output on a regular basis, the result for too many of us is gaining weight.

We need to adapt our lifestyle to our high-caloric diet and lack of exercise. It's become very important to catch bursts of physical activity wherever we can to increase our energy output. (See the following chapter for more information on exercise.)

While you work on increasing your energy output, the glycemic index can help you select the best foods to balance your intake. Its high carbohydrate basis ensures a filling diet that isn't packed with calories.

◀ 8 ▶

THE BENEFITS OF LIVING
AN ACTIVE LIFE

$\mathcal{D}$IET ISN'T THE only way to manage diabetes. Because the disease stays with you for the rest of your life, taking good care of yourself requires adopting a few healthy lifestyle habits that must last a lifetime.

A multitude of changes in our living habits now means that in both work and recreation we are more sedentary than ever. Our physical activity levels are now so low that we take in more calories than we burn off, causing us to gain weight. Luckily, exercise is our ticket back to healthy living.

Regular physical activity can reduce our blood sugar levels, lower our risk of heart and blood vessel disease, lower high blood pressure, increase stamina, reduce stress and help us relax. It's a good idea for all of us.

■

To lose weight you need to eat fewer calories and burn
more calories—and that means getting regular exercise
and leading a more active lifestyle.

■

THE BENEFITS OF EXERCISE

Most people could tell you at least one health benefit of
exercise (reduces blood pressure, lowers the risk of heart
disease, improves circulation, increases stamina, flexibil-
ity and strength), but the most motivating aspect of exercise is feeling so good about yourself for doing it.

Exercise speeds up our metabolic rate. By increasing
our caloric expenditure, exercise helps to balance our
sometimes excessive caloric intake from food.

More movement makes our muscles better at using
fat as a source of fuel. By improving the way insulin
works, exercise increases the amount of fat we burn.

A low-GI diet has the same effect. Low-GI foods
reduce the amount of insulin we need, which makes fat
easier to burn and harder to store. Since it's body fat that
you want to get rid of when you lose weight, exercise in
combination with a low-GI diet makes a lot of sense!

HOW TO GET MOVING

Getting more exercise doesn't necessarily mean daily aer-
obics classes and jogging around the block (although this

is great if you want to do it). What it does mean is moving more in everyday living. It's the day-to-day things we do— shopping, ironing, chasing kids, walking from the train station—where we spend the bulk of our energy.

Since so much of our lifestyle is designed now to reduce our physical exertion, it's become very important to catch bursts of physical activity wherever we can, to increase our energy output. It may mean using the stairs instead of the elevator, taking a 10-minute walk at lunch time, trotting on a treadmill while you watch the news or talk on the telephone, walking to the grocery store to get the Sunday paper, hiding the remote control, parking a half mile from work, or taking the dog for a walk each night. Whatever it means, do it. Even housework burns calories!

How Exercise Keeps Burning Calories, Even When You Are at Rest

THE EFFECT OF exercise doesn't stop when you do. People who exercise have higher metabolic rates, so their bodies continue to burn more calories every minute, even when they're asleep!

Besides increasing the incidental activity, you will also benefit from some planned aerobic activity, which causes you to breathe more heavily and makes your heart beat faster. Walking, cycling, swimming, and stair climbing are just a few examples. You'll need to accumulate a total of at least 30 minutes of this type of activity five to six days a week.

Remember that reduction in body weight takes time. Even after you've made changes in your exercise habits, your weight may not be any different on the scale. (This is particularly true for women, whose bodies tend to adapt to increased caloric expenditure.)

Whatever it takes for you to burn more calories, do it. Try to regard movement as an opportunity to improve your physical well-being—not as an inconvenience.

USING THE GLYCEMIC INDEX WHEN YOU EXERCISE

We're talking about the everyday sort of moderate exercise that all of us should be doing. If you train physically hard a number of days a week and perhaps compete in sports you should read *The Glucose Revolution Pocket Guide to Sports Nutrition*.

It is sometimes necessary with diabetes to eat extra carbohydrate when you exercise depending on the type of diabetes you have and the type and amount of medication you take. Often, you won't want to increase your food intake—because the exercise is intended to burn off some earlier overconsumption! (For people with type 1 diabetes, remember this will only work if you have enough insulin in your body and your blood sugars aren't too high to start with.)

You may need extra carbohydrate before you exercise, or, if the exercise is prolonged over an hour or more, you may need extra carbohydrate while you exercise, too. Whether or not you need to eat extra, and how much to take, depends on your blood sugar level before, during, and after the exercise, and how your body responds to the exercise—all of which you learn from experience. Discuss your situation and how best to manage it with a dietitian, diabetes educator or doctor.

If you need to eat immediately before exercise to bring your blood sugar up during exercise, it makes sense to eat some high-GI carbohydrate, such as a slice of regular bread, a couple of cookies, or a ripe banana.

If you plan to eat your last meal or snack one to two hours before your exercise, it makes sense to eat a low-GI meal to sustain you through the exercise, such as a sandwich made with low-GI bread, lowfat protein such as turkey breast or boiled ham, a container of yogurt, or an apple.

If you need to eat something quickly after or during exercise to restore your blood sugar level, use high-GI food—crispbread or rice cakes, a bowl of corn flakes or Rice Krispies, or a slice of watermelon, for example.

> NOTE: Always remember to measure your blood sugar when you exercise to assess your body's response and judge your carbohydrate needs.

■

**Exercise makes our muscles better
at using fat as a source of fuel.**

■

8 WAYS TO MAKE EXERCISE WORK FOR YOU

Your exercise routine will bring you lots of benefits if you can:

1. appreciate its benefits
2. enjoy doing it
3. feel good about your ability to exercise
4. make it a normal part of your day
5. keep it inexpensive
6. make it accessible
7. stay safe while doing it
8. do it with someone

◆ 9 ◆

YOUR NUTRIENT COUNTER

*T*O MEET YOUR average daily nutrient requirements you need to eat a certain amount of different types of foods. If you are trying to reduce your caloric intake there is still a minimum amount of certain foods that you should be eating each day. These are:

BREADS/CEREALS/AND GRAIN FOODS—
SIX SERVINGS OR MORE

One serving means:
▶ One bowl breakfast cereal (1 oz)
▶ ½ cup cooked pasta or rice
▶ ½ cup cooked grain such as barley or wheat
▶ One slice bread
▶ One half roll or muffin

VEGETABLES—THREE SERVINGS

One serving means:
- One medium potato (about 5 oz)
- ½ cup cooked vegetables such as broccoli or carrot (2 oz)
- 1 cup raw leafy vegetables, such as lettuce

FRUIT—TWO TO FOUR SERVINGS

One serving means:
- One medium orange (7 oz)
- One medium apple (5 oz)
- ½ cup strawberries (4 oz)

DAIRY FOODS—TWO SERVINGS

One serving means:
- 8 ounces low fat milk
- 1½ ounces low-fat cheese
- 8 ounces low-fat yogurt

MEAT AND ALTERNATIVES—TWO SERVINGS

One serving means:
- 3 ounces cooked lean beef, veal, lamb or pork
- 3 ounces lean chicken (cooked, excluding bone)
- 3 ounces fish (cooked, excluding bone)
- Two eggs
- ½ cup cooked beans

◀ 10 ▶

HOW WELL ARE YOU
EATING NOW?

*Y*OU CAN CHECK the nutritional quality of your diet yourself; all you need is a record of your usual food intake. It is ideal if you can keep a food diary of everything you eat and drink for three to five days and use this for your assessment. Remember you have to eat as freely as you normally do, and write down everything—otherwise you're only cheating yourself!

Once you have your total food intake record complete, use the following serving size guidelines to check whether you have a balanced intake. The checklists on the following pages can be used to assess your carbohydrate and fat intake.

DO YOU EAT ENOUGH CARBOHYDRATE?

Looking at your diet record and using the serving size guide below, estimate the number of servings of carbohydrate foods you had each day. For example, if you had a banana, two slices of bread, and a medium potato, this counts as four servings of carbohydrate.

CARBOHYDRATE FOOD	ONE SERVING IS	HOW MANY DID YOU EAT?
Bread	one slice	
Low GI:		
100% stoneground whole wheat, pumpernickel, sourdough, rye		
High GI:		
White, Italian, baguette		
Beverages	about ¾ cup (6 oz)	
Low GI:		
Apple, tomato, grapefruit juice		
High GI:		
Cranberry juice cocktail, Gatorade		
Cooked breakfast cereals	½ cup cooked cereal	
Low GI:		
Old-fashioned oats, apple and cinnamon hot cereal, ConAgra		
High GI:		
Instant Cream of Wheat, instant oatmeal		
Fruit	a handful or one medium piece	
Low GI:		
Apples, bananas, oranges, grapes, peaches, strawberries		
High GI:		
Canned fruit cocktail, pineapple, watermelon		
Legumes	½ cup, cooked	
Low GI:		
Lentils; kidney, navy, pinto, lima beans		

CARBOHYDRATE FOOD	ONE SERVING IS	HOW MANY DID YOU EAT?
Muffins, rolls	one half roll, muffin, or small bagel	
Low GI:		
Apple muffin, chocolate-butterscotch muffin		
High GI:		
English muffin, bagel, doughnut		
Noodles and rice	½ cup, cooked	
Low GI:		
Fettuccine, macaroni, tortellini		
High GI:		
Gnocchi, jasmine rice, arborio (risotto) rice		
Ready-to-eat breakfast cereals	1-oz bowl	
Low GI:		
Kellogg's All-Bran, Complete Bran Flakes		
High GI:		
Cheerios, Grapenuts, Rice Krispies		
Starchy vegetables	½ cup cooked or 1 cup raw	
Low GI:		
Sweet potato, squash, peas		
High GI:		
Mashed potato, pumpkin, frozen French fries		
Total:		

Average the number of servings over all the days to come up with a daily average.

Low-GI Eating

Low-GI eating means making a move back to the high carbohydrate foods that are staples in many parts of the world, especially whole grains (barley, oats, dried peas, and beans) in combination with breads, pasta, vegetables, fruits, and certain types of rice.

HOW DID YOUR SERVINGS RATE?

- Fewer than four servings a day: Poor.
- Between four and eight servings a day:
  Fair, but you need to eat a lot more.
- Between nine and twelve servings a day:
  Good, could need more if you are hungry.
- Between thirteen and sixteen servings a day:
  Great—this should meet the needs of most people.

HOW DID YOUR GI VALUES RATE?

- Fewer than four low-GI foods a day: Poor.
- Between four and eight low-GI foods a day:
  Fair, but you need to eat a lot more low-GI foods.
- Between nine and twelve low-GI foods a day:
  Good, but try to add more of these food choices.
- Between thirteen and sixteen low-GI foods a day:
  Great—you're eating a low-GI diet.

IS YOUR DIET TOO HIGH IN FAT?

Use this fat counter to tally up how much fat your diet
contains. Do a tally for each day and then take an average. Using this fat counter, you will need to compare
the serving size listed with your serving size and multiply the grams of fat up or down to match your serving
size. For example, if you estimate you might consume 2
cups of regular milk in a day, this supplies you with 16
grams of fat.

FOOD	FAT CONTENT (GRAMS)	HOW MUCH DID YOU EAT?
Dairy Foods		
Milk (8 oz) 1 cup		
whole	8	
2%	5	
nonfat	0	
Yogurt (8 oz)		
whole milk	7	
nonfat	0	
Ice cream, two scoops (1 cup)		
regular	15	
low fat	3	
fat free	0	
Cheese		
American, block cheese, 1-oz slice	9	
reduced fat American cheese, 1-oz slice	7	
low fat slices (per slice)	3	
cottage, small curd, 2 tbsps	3	
ricotta, whole milk, 2 tbsps	2	
Cream, 1 tbsp		
heavy	6	
light	5	
Sour cream, 1 tbsp		
regular	3	
light	1	
Fats and Oils		
Butter, 1 tsp	4	
Oil, any type, 1 tbsp (½ oz)	14	
Cooking spray, per spray	0	
Mayonnaise, 1 tbsp	11	
Salad dressing, 1 tbsp	6	
Meat		
Beef		
steak, flank, lean only, 3½ oz	10	
ground beef, extra-lean, 1 cup, 3½ oz, cooked, drained	16	
sausage, frankfurter, grilled, 2 oz	16	
top sirloin, lean only, 3½ oz	8	
Lamb		

rib chop, grilled, lean only, 3½ oz	10
leg, roasted, lean only, 3½ oz	7
loin chop, grilled, lean only, 3½ oz	8
Pork	
bacon, three strips, panfried	9
ham, one slice, leg, lean, 3½ oz	5
steak, lean only, 3½ oz	4
leg, roasted, lean only, 3½ oz	9
loin chop, lean only, 3½ oz	4
Chicken	
breast, skinless, 3 oz	4
drumstick, skinless, 2 oz	3
thigh, skinless, 2 oz	6
one half barbecued chicken (including skin)	30
Fish	
one grilled average-sized fish fillet, 4 oz	1
salmon, 3 oz	3
four frozen fish sticks, baked	14
two frozen fish fillets, batter-dipped, oven-baked, 6 oz	
regular	26
light	10

Snack Foods

Chocolate bar, Hershey's, 1½ oz	13
Potato chips, 1-oz bag	10
Corn chips, 1-oz bag	10
Peanuts, ½ cups, (2½ oz)	35
French fries, twenty-five pieces	20
Medium pizza, cheese, two slices,	22
Apple pie, snack size	15
Popcorn, fat and salt added, 3 cups	9

Total:

HOW DID YOU RATE?

- Less than 40 grams: Excellent. 30 to 40 grams of fat per day is recommended for those people trying to lose weight.
- 41 to 60 grams: Good. A fat intake in this range is recommended for most adult men and women.
- 61 to 80 grams: Acceptable if you are very active (doing hard physical work or athletic training). It is probably too much if you are trying to lose weight.
- More than 80 grams: You're probably eating too much fat, unless you're Superman or Superwoman!

NOTE: The foods in this list have not been categorized as high or low GI since, with the exception of the snack foods, all other entries contain little or no carbohydrate, and thus are not ranked by the glycemic index.

◀ **11** ▶

SECRETS TO LOW-GI
SNACKING

*M*ANY PEOPLE WITH diabetes need between-meal snacks to keep their blood sugar levels from dipping too low. The glycemic index is especially important when you eat carbohydrate by itself and not as part of a mixed meal, because carbohydrate tends to have a stronger effect on our blood sugar level when it is eaten alone.

When choosing a between-meal bite, pick a low-fat snack with a low glycemic index. For example, an apple with a glycemic index of 38 is better than a slice of white bread with a glycemic index of around 70, because it will cause a smaller jump in blood sugar levels and quiet the stomach growls until the next meal.

New evidence suggests that people who graze, eating small amounts of food throughout the day at frequent intervals, may actually be doing themselves a favor. Spreading the food out over longer periods of time will flatten out the peaks and valleys of blood glucose levels. So, snacking may be a good idea if you have diabetes—as long as you don't overeat and gain weight. Snack calories are not *extra* calories—they are either taken from the prior meal or from the upcoming one.

Some snack foods with a very low glycemic index (such as peanuts, at 14) have a very high fat content. As an occasional snack they are fine, especially because their fat is heart-healthy. Just don't go overboard. Seven nuts is a healthy portion—it may seem very small at first, but you'll soon find the sustaining power in these energy-filled snack choices.

SEVENTEEN SUSTAINING SNACKS

- an apple
- oat bran muffin
- dried apricots
- a mini can of baked beans
- a small bowl of cherries
- ice cream (low fat) in a cone
- milk, milkshake or smoothie (low fat, of course)
- up to three oatmeal cookies
- an orange
- ¼ cup dried fruit and nut fruit mix
- pita bread spread with apple butter
- handful of sourdough pretzel nuggets
- one or two slices of raisin toast
- half a whole grain bread sandwich with your favorite filling
- a small bowl of bran flakes with skim milk
- one or two graham crackers with one tablespoon natural peanut butter
- 6–8 ounces of light yogurt

FIVE SNACKING TIPS

- It is important to include at least two servings of dairy foods each day for your calcium needs. A low-fat milkshake, one or two scoops of low-fat ice cream or yogurt, fat free cooked pudding, or reduced-fat cheese can boost your daily calcium intake.

- If you like whole grain breads, an extra slice makes a very good choice for a snack. Other snacks can include toasted sourdough English muffin halves, a whole grain waffle or a slice of raisin bread with a little butter, peanut butter, or apple butter.

- Fruit is always a low calorie option for snacks. You should try to consume at least three servings a day. It may be helpful to prepare fruit in advance to make it accessible for quick and easy eating.

- Whole grain crackers are a low-calorie snack if you want something dry and crunchy. Popcorn, sourdough pretzel nuggets, or a small handful of dry-roasted nuts are other good alternatives.

- Keep vegetables (such as celery and carrot sticks, baby tomatoes, florets of blanched cauliflower or broccoli) readily available for quick and easy snacking.

◀ 12 ▶

STOCKING YOUR
LOW-GI PANTRY

WHAT TO KEEP ON YOUR COUNTER

Breads
- 100% stoneground whole-wheat
- 100% stoneground whole-wheat pita
- chapati (Baisen)
- Healthy Choice Hearty 7 Grain
- Natural Ovens 100% Whole Grain**
- Natural Ovens Happiness Raisin Pecan**
- Natural Ovens Hunger Filler**
- Natural Ovens Natural Wheat
- Natural Ovens Nutty Natural, whole grain**
- Natural Ovens Multi-Grain Stay Trim, whole grain**
- rye
- sourdough

**Natural Ovens breads are available in the United States through mail order. See "For More Information" on page 169 for ordering information.

- sourdough rye
- Spelt, multi-grain
- whole grain pumpernickel

WHAT TO KEEP IN YOUR PANTRY

Breakfast cereals

- ConAgra apple and cinnamon hot cereal
- Kellogg's All-Bran
- Kellogg's All-Bran with Extra Fiber™
- Kellogg's Bran Buds
- Kellogg's Bran Buds with Psyllium™
- Kellogg's Multi-Bran Chex™
- Kellogg's Complete Bran Flakes
- Kellogg's Just Right
- Kellogg's Raisin Bran
- muesli (low-fat varieties, read the labels)
- oat bran
- rice bran
- rolled or old-fashioned oats

Cookies and Cakes

- apple cinnamon muffin, from mix*
- Arrowroot cookies
- banana bread
- chocolate cake with chocolate frosting
- FIFTY50 Hearty Oatmeal cookies
- FIFTY50 sugar free oatmeal cookies
- FIFTY50 vanilla creme-filled wafers
- oatmeal cookies

*Contains fat in excess of American Heart Association Guidelines.
Use only once in a while and in small amounts.

- pound cake
- shortbread cookies
- Social Tea™ biscuits
- sponge cake
- vanilla cake

Rices and Grains

- barley, cracked
- barley, pearled
- basmati rice, brown or long-grain rice
- brown rice
- buckwheat
- buchwheat groats
- bulgur
- dried noodles
- dried pasta
- pasta of various shapes and flavors
- pearled barley
- rolled oats
- Uncle Ben's Cajun Style rice
- Uncle Ben's Original Converted™ rice
- Uncle Ben's Long Grain and Wild rice

Legumes

- a variety of canned legumes (kidney beans, mixed beans, baked beans, lentils, chickpeas, black beans, pinto beans, butter beans, chana dal)
- cooked lentils (red or brown), chickpeas, split peas
- dried lentils, chickpeas, cannellini beans

Spices, sauces, and condiments

- black pepper
- bottled pasta sauces

- bottled spices such as ginger, chili, and garlic
- bottled vegetables such as sun-dried tomatoes, roasted eggplant or peppers, marinated artichoke, and mushrooms
- canned corn, tomatoes, asparagus, peas, and mushrooms
- canned evaporated skim milk
- canned new potatoes
- canned peaches, pears, and apples
- canned tuna or sardines in spring water, canned salmon
- canola oil
- capers, olives, and anchovies
- curry paste
- dried fruits, including raisins, apricots, fruit medley, prunes
- extra virgin olive oil
- honey
- jarred chutneys
- JELL-O Brand Cook & Serve Fat Free Sugar Free Pudding & Pie Filling™
- low fat salad dressings
- low sodium bouillon
- mustard seed
- sauces (such as soy, chili, oyster, hoisin, teriyaki, low sodium Worcestershire)
- sesame oil
- shelf-stable skim milk or skim milk powder
- soup stocks
- spices, such as ground cumin, garlic powder, curry powder, mustard, cinnamon, nutmeg, catsup, freshly ground pepper, hot pepper, turmeric, dried oregano, basil, thyme, and parsley

- tomato paste and tomato puree
- vinegar

WHAT TO KEEP IN YOUR FRIDGE

- apples
- canned peaches, pears, apples
- cherries
- corn
- dried fruits, such as dried apricots, fruit medley, prunes
- fresh vegetables, especially those in season
- grapefruit
- grapes
- kiwi
- oranges
- peaches
- pears
- peas
- plums
- sweet potatoes or yams

Miscellaneous
- fresh pasta or noodles

Dairy products
- cheese: Low-fat processed slices, reduced-fat Swiss (such as Jarlsberg Light), grated Parmesan, 1% or 2% cottage, or part skim ricotta cheese
- eggs
- frozen low-fat yogurt, sorbet, gelato
- light fruited yogurt
- non-fat plain yogurt

- skim or 1% milk

WHAT TO KEEP IN YOUR FREEZER

- baby beans
- frozen berries and melon balls
- low-fat ice cream
- frozen vegetables

Hypoglycemia: the Exception to the Low GI Rule

IF YOU TAKE insulin or pills to treat diabetes, your blood sugar level may sometimes fall below 70, which is the lower end of the normal range. When this happens you might feel hungry, shaky, or sweaty and be unable to think clearly. This is called low blood sugar or "hypoglycemia."

Hypoglycemia is a potentially dangerous situation and must be treated right away by eating some carbohydrate food. In this case you should pick a carbohydrate with a high glycemic index because you need to increase your blood sugar quickly. Jelly beans (GI value of 80) are a good choice. If you are not due for your next meal or snack, you should also have some low-GI carbohydrate (an apple, for example), to keep your blood sugar from falling again until you next eat.

■

**Glucose tablets or jelly beans
are good choices for treating low blood sugar.**

■

◀ 13 ▶

LOW GI EATING MADE EASY

*A*LTHOUGH THERE ARE bad *diets*, no individual food is bad, especially when it comes to the glycemic index. Eating the low-GI way means eating a variety of foods—possibly a wider variety than you are already eating.

Usually we eat a combination of carbohydrate foods, such as sandwiches and fruit, pasta and bread, cereal and toast, potatoes and corn. The glycemic index of a meal consisting of a mixture of carbohydrate foods is a weighted average of the glycemic index of the carbohydrate foods. The weighting is based on the proportion of the total carbohydrate contributed by each food. Studies show that when a food with a high glycemic index is combined with a food with a low glycemic index the complete meal has an intermediate glycemic index.

As with calories, the GI value is not precise. The glycemic index gives you a guide to help you lower the glycemic index of your day, and just one simple change can make a big difference. Look at the following ideas for the meals in your day and see how you could lower the glycemic index of your diet.

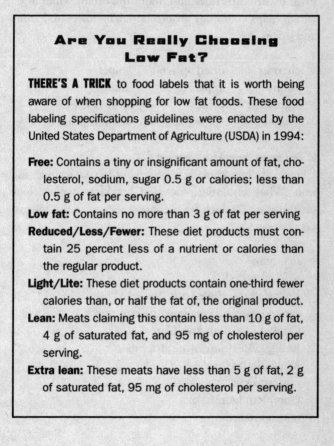

Are You Really Choosing Low Fat?

THERE'S A TRICK to food labels that it is worth being aware of when shopping for low fat foods. These food labeling specifications guidelines were enacted by the United States Department of Agriculture (USDA) in 1994:

Free: Contains a tiny or insignificant amount of fat, cholesterol, sodium, sugar 0.5 g or calories; less than 0.5 g of fat per serving.

Low fat: Contains no more than 3 g of fat per serving

Reduced/Less/Fewer: These diet products must contain 25 percent less of a nutrient or calories than the regular product.

Light/Lite: These diet products contain one-third fewer calories than, or half the fat of, the original product.

Lean: Meats claiming this contain less than 10 g of fat, 4 g of saturated fat, and 95 mg of cholesterol per serving.

Extra lean: These meats have less than 5 g of fat, 2 g of saturated fat, 95 mg of cholesterol per serving.

BREAKFAST BASICS

1. Include some fruit

Fruit contributes fiber and, more important, vitamin C, which helps your body absorb iron. The lowest-GI fruits and juices are:

cherries	dried apricots	grapes
plums	apples	oranges
grapefruit	pears	strawberries
peaches	apple juice	grapefruit juice

2. Try some breakfast cereal

Cereals are important as a source of fiber, vitamin B, and iron. When choosing processed breakfast cereals, look for those with a high fiber content. Some of the lowest-GI cereals are:

rice bran
toasted muesli
Kellog's Bran Buds with Psyllium™
cooked oatmeal (made with skim milk)
Quaker Oat Bran Hot Cereal
Kellog's All-Bran with Extra Fiber™
Multi-Bran Chex™
raw oat bran
Complete bran flakes
natural muesli

3. Add milk or yogurt

Low-fat milks and yogurts can make a valuable contribution to your daily calcium intake when you include them at breakfast. All have a low glycemic index, and

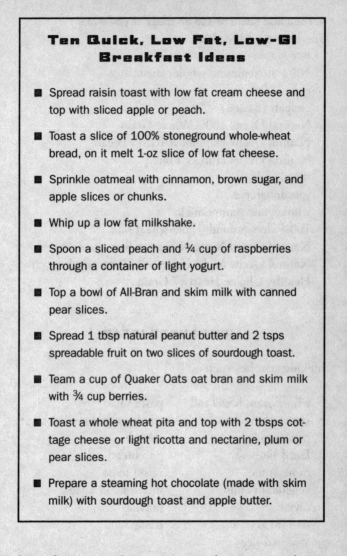

Ten Quick, Low Fat, Low-GI Breakfast Ideas

■ Spread raisin toast with low fat cream cheese and top with sliced apple or peach.

■ Toast a slice of 100% stoneground whole-wheat bread, on it melt 1-oz slice of low fat cheese.

■ Sprinkle oatmeal with cinnamon, brown sugar, and apple slices or chunks.

■ Whip up a low fat milkshake.

■ Spoon a sliced peach and ¼ cup of raspberries through a container of light yogurt.

■ Top a bowl of All-Bran and skim milk with canned pear slices.

■ Spread 1 tbsp natural peanut butter and 2 tsps spreadable fruit on two slices of sourdough toast.

■ Team a cup of Quaker Oats oat bran and skim milk with ¾ cup berries.

■ Toast a whole wheat pita and top with 2 tbsps cottage cheese or light ricotta and nectarine, plum or pear slices.

■ Prepare a steaming hot chocolate (made with skim milk) with sourdough toast and apple butter.

lower fat varieties have just as much, or more, calcium as whole milk.

4. Then add some bread or toast, if you'd like

The lowest-GI breads are:

100% stoneground whole-wheat
rye
chapati (Baisen)
Natural Ovens 100% Whole-Grain
Natural Ovens Happiness Raisin Pecan
Natural Ovens Hunger Filler
sourdough
sourdough rye
whole grain pumpernickel
100% stoneground whole-wheat pita
Natural Ovens Nutty Natural, whole grain
Natural Ovens Multi-Grain Stay Trim, whole-grain
Healthy Choice Hearty 7 Grain

LIGHT LUNCH IDEAS

Include starches such as:

whole-grain bread roll
sweet corn
pea soup
lentil soup
minestrone
vegetarian chili
ravioli
rice salad
steamed rice

pasta salad
whole-grain bread or toast
tabouli
pita bread
raisin toast
mixed bean salad
noodles
pasta

1. Base your light meals on carbohydrate

2. Include some high protein foods, such as:
    boiled ham, fresh turkey or chicken breast,
       lean roast beef
    reduced fat cheese
    small can of tuna, salmon, or sardines
    natural, no-salt-added peanut butter and all-fruit
       jelly or fruit butter
    hard-boiled egg or vegetable omelet

3. Always include a hardy portion of vegetables. Here are some suggestions:
    broccoli
    shredded cabbage
    grated carrot
    cauliflower florets
    celery sticks
    chard
    cucumber
    eggplant
    mushrooms
    pepper strips
    salad greens
    sliced shallots or onions,
    snow peas
    spinach
    sprouts
    sun dried tomatoes
    cherry, grape, or plum tomatoes
    zucchini

4. And round it off with fruit

Ten Low-GI Lunches on the Go

1. Pita with hummus and tomatoes or broccoli
2. Pasta with pesto, sun dried tomatoes, and part skim ricotta
3. Grilled ham, cheese, and tomato sandwich on sourdough rye
4. Melted cheese and tomato sandwich on 100% stoneground whole wheat bread
5. 8 oz light yogurt, 1½ cups fresh fruit salad, 2–3 graham crackers
6. Large mixed salad with beans, olives, and sunflower seeds
7. Chunky vegetable soup with barley and beans, and a piece of fruit
8. Veggie burger with salsa and grilled vegetables on 100% whole wheat sandwich bun
9. Smoked salmon and avocado slices on pumpernickel bread
10. A fruit smoothie and high fiber blueberry oat bran muffin

---

◀ 14 ▶

MASTERING LOW-GI MEALS

JUST ONE OF the advantages of a low GI diet is the tremendous variety of foods it offers. You can eat just about anything you want—including dessert! Let the ideas below jump-start your menu-planning creativity.

1. FIRST CHOOSE THE CARBOHYDRATE

Which will it be? A new or sweet potato? Basmati or Uncle Ben's Original Converted Rice? A type of pasta? A grain, such as cracked wheat or barley? Chickpeas, lentils, or beans? Or a combination? Could you add some bread or corn?

2. ADD VEGETABLES—AND LOTS OF THEM

Fresh, frozen, or canned—the more the merrier.

artichokes	eggplant	radishes
asparagus	fennel	salad greens
beans	leeks	squash
bok choy	mushrooms	tomatoes
brussels sprouts	okra	zucchini
cabbage	onions	
carrots	peas	
cauliflower	pea pods	
celery	peppers	

3. NOW, JUST A LITTLE PROTEIN FOR FLAVOR AND TEXTURE

Remember, you don't need much—some slivers of beef to stir fry, a sprinkle of tasty cheese, strips of ham, a dollop of ricotta, a tender chicken breast, slices of salmon, a couple of eggs, a handful of nuts, or use the protein found in your grains and legumes.

4. THINK TWICE ABOUT USING ANY FAT

Check that you are using a healthy type (monounsaturated or polyunsaturated), such as canola or olive oil.

Ten Low GI Dinner Ideas

1. Spaghetti with meatballs and a large mixed salad
2. Fish fillet stuffed with fresh herbs, tomatoes, and onions, baked in foil; serve with heavy grain bread roll, steamed vegetables, or large mixed salad
3. Stir-fried shrimp, scallops, beef, or chicken, and vegetables over basmati rice or lo mein noodles
4. Grilled steak with grilled vegetables and an ear of corn
5. Omelet with ham, cheese, vegetables, beans, or salsa filling; serve with rice pilaf and asparagus spears
6. Spinach or cheese tortellini, fresh tomato sauce, and steamed garden vegetable medley
7. Chicken or tuna casserole, with mixed vegetables and new potatoes
8. Meat or vegetarian lasagna served with a large mixed salad
9. Barbecued chicken, steamed corn and tomato, onion, and cucumber salad
10. Beef, chicken, or bean soft tortilla topped with salsa, served with a large mixed salad

DESSERTS: A LOW GI FINISH

Although often overlooked, desserts can make a valuable contribution to your daily calcium and vitamin C intake when they are based on low fat dairy foods and fruits. Recipes incorporating fruit for sweetness will have more fiber and lower GI values than recipes with sugar. What's more, desserts are usually carbohydrate rich, which means they help top-up our satiety center, signifying the completion of eating and reducing the tendency for late night nibbles.

If you don't have time to prepare a dessert, why not simply serve a bowl of seasonal fruit?

apples	oranges
apricots	papaya
bananas	peaches
blueberries	pears
cantaloupe	persimmons
cherries	plums
grapefruit	prunes
grapes	quinces
honeydew melon	raspberries
kiwi	rhubarb
mandarins	star fruit
mangoes	strawberries
nectarines	

■

A rule of thumb:
High GI food + Low GI food = Intermediate GI meal

■

Ten Quick and Easy Low GI Desserts

1. Low-fat ice cream and strawberries
2. Baked apple stuffed with dried cranberries
3. Fresh fruit salad—sprinkle of granola or nuts topped with light yogurt
4. Fruit crisp (for topping use low fat granola, crumbled bran flakes, or oats, and a little melted butter and honey)
5. Cooked low-fat pudding
6. Warmed canned peach or pear slices (unsweetened)—sprinkle with cardamom and top with with a dollop of Cool Whip Lite
7. Struedel—wrap sliced apples, raisins, currants and spice, in a sheet of filo pastry (brushed with milk, not fat) and bake
8. Citrus fruit medley in a brandied honey sauce
9. Homemade chunky applesauce and graham crackers
10. Low-fat fruit mousse

◀ 15 ▶

A WEEK OF LOW GI MENUS

$\mathcal{J}$HIS WEEK OF menus shows you how to eat a healthy, low-GI diet. Use the menus for ideas to make sure you eat low fat, high carbohydrate, low-GI meals every day.

We have included between-meal snacks in most of the menus as people who take medication (including insulin) to help control their diabetes generally need them. While not everyone with diabetes has to eat between meals, snacks can be a normal part of a healthy diet.

We have analyzed each menu to estimate its calories and the amount of fat, carbohydrate and fiber. We have also calculated the GI values. By emphasizing low-GI foods, we have created menus with predicted low GI numbers, that is, below 55. Here are some points to consider.

1. CALORIES

Calories are a measure of the total amount of energy available from a food. Each day you require a certain amount of calories to fuel your body. The younger and more active you are the more energy you need. If you want to lose weight, you may need to reduce your calorie intake. The calorie levels of these menus are reasonably low and represent a minimum requirement for most people.

2. FAT

People with diabetes are advised to eat a low fat diet. The menus are examples of low fat meals if you use skim milk and minimal amounts of butter and other fats and oils when preparing them. If you are trying to lose weight, aim for a fat intake of 30–50 grams per day. Remember, such low fat diets are not recommended for young children.

3. CARBOHYDRATE

These menus are all high in carbohydrate, deriving about half the total calories from that nutrient. For a small eater, this represents about 150 to 200 grams of carbohydrate per day. The more active you are the more carbohydrate you need. Note that 150 to 200 grams of carbohydrate equates to 10 to 13 carbohydrate exchanges (for people who use that system).

4. FIBER

Guidelines suggest you need at least 30 grams of fiber each day. This is often difficult to achieve on a low calorie intake without eating a high fiber cereal every morning. The fiber content of these menus varies from 20 to 40 grams per day, giving a daily average of 30 grams.

FIVE LITTLE TIPS
THAT MAKE A BIG DIFFERENCE

- Think of carbohydrate foods as the number-one priority in your meals.
- Change a dietary staple (such as bread) to a low-GI staple to lower the overall glycemic index of your meals.
- Get in touch with your true appetite and use it to guide the amount of food you eat. Low-fat, high-fiber, low-GI foods fill you up best.
- Try to eat at least two low GI meals each day.
- Mix high-GI foods with low-GI foods in your meals—the combination will give an overall intermediate glycemic index.

We understand that the portions listed in these menus may seem small—at least at first. But the good news is, as long as you're moving *toward* eating smaller portions (and we're showing you the appropriate portion sizes for the calories), you'll be making progress. The proof of that progress will show up in your weight and in your blood sugar, cholesterol, and blood pressure numbers.

MONDAY

GI:	47
Total Energy:	1531 cal
Fat:	31 g
Carbohydrate:	231 g
Fiber:	40 g

■

Breakfast: Cereal and toast
Prepare ½ cup Raisin Bran with ½ cup 1% milk, one slice of 100% stoneground whole-wheat bread (toasted), with 1 tablespoon of light margarine, and 1 teaspoon of spreadable fruit.

Morning snack: An apple

Lunch: Tuna sandwich and salad
Combine ½ cup of canned tuna with a little onion, parsley, and 1 tablespoon low-fat mayonnaise. Place tuna and thin tomato slices between 2 slices of 100% stoneground whole-wheat bread and have it with 1 cup of mixed-bean salad and salad greens.

Afternoon snack: One cup of grapes (3 oz)

Dinner: Grilled steak and vegetables

Evening snack: An 8-ounce container of light fruited yogurt

TUESDAY

GI:	44
Total Energy:	1562 cal
Fat:	38 g
Carbohydrate:	221 g
Fiber:	28 g

■

Breakfast: Oatmeal
Cook ½ cup old-fashioned oats with ½ cup water and ½ cup skim milk. Serve with a teaspoon of brown sugar or honey, or four peach slices.

Morning snack: An orange

Lunch: A sandwich on the run
Cheese and arugula in a whole-wheat pita.

Afternoon snack: An 8-ounce container of light fruited yogurt

Dinner: Spaghetti and meat sauce
Add ¾ cup of meat sauce to about 1 cup of spaghetti and sprinkle with a teaspoon of grated Parmesan cheese. Include a large tossed salad with fat-free dressing and a glass of red wine if desired. For dessert, help yourself to a large baked apple sprinkled with cinnamon.

Evening snack: A bunch of grapes

WEDNESDAY

GI:	44
Total Energy:	1603 cal
Fat:	43 g
Carbohydrate:	218 g
Fiber:	36 g

■

Breakfast: Cereal, fruit and toast
Prepare ½ cup All Bran with ½ cup unsweetened canned peaches and ¾ cup skim milk, and one slice of 100% stoneground whole-wheat toast with 1 teaspoon natural peanut butter.

Morning snack: Two oatmeal cookies and ¾ cup skim milk

Lunch: A toasted ham sandwich
Place 2 ounces ham and tomato on two slices toasted pumpernickel bread. Finish with an apple.

Afternoon snack: An orange

Dinner: Stir fry and rice
Stir-fry flank steak strips (about 3½ oz raw weight) and a combination of at least 1 cup vegetables (such as broccoli, zucchini, shallots, cabbage), adding 1 tablespoon peanut oil, soy sauce, ginger, garlic, etc. to flavor. Serve with a cup of boiled rice such as basmati or Uncle Ben's Converted Rice.

Evening snack: A juicy peach or other fresh fruit in season

THURSDAY

GI:	46
Total Energy:	1464 cal
Fat:	24 g
Carbohydrate:	231 g
Fiber:	38 g

■

Breakfast: Muesli, fruit, and yogurt
   Combine ⅔ cup Swiss-style muesli with 6 ounces
   light fruited yogurt and a fresh sliced pear.
Morning snack: Two Ryvita with 1 tablespoon natural
   peanut butter
Lunch: A filled spud
   Microwave a large 6-ounce sweet potato in its skin.
   Slice off the top, scoop out the middle, mix the potato
   with 1 tablespoon each of cottage cheese or reduced-
   fat goat cheese, diced ham, reduced-fat cheddar
   cheese, and a sprinkle of chopped scallions. Stuff this
   mixture into the potato skin and reheat.
Afternoon snack: One cup low fat chocolate milk
Dinner: Mexican beef and beans
   Fill a 2-ounce soft tortilla with ½ cup stir-fried kidney
   beans, peppers, onions, tomatoes, and 3 ounces of
   beef strips. Add a sprinkle of reduced-fat cheddar
   cheese. Roll up or fold the tortilla. Heat in a warmed
   oven for 5 minutes.
Evening snack: A large apple

FRIDAY

GI:	48
Total Energy:	1496 cal
Fat:	28 g
Carbohydrate:	225 g
Fiber:	25 g

■

Breakfast: Peach smoothie and graham crackers

Whip up a medium peach (fresh, frozen, or canned), 4 ounces light yogurt, 4 ounces skim milk, and 1 tablespoon honey in a blender to make a quick liquid breakfast. Serve with four graham cracker squares. Save any leftovers for a morning snack.

Lunch: Grilled cheese and tomato

Cover 2 slices of sourdough bread each with two or three thin tomato slices and 1 ounce low-fat cheddar cheese. Heat in toaster oven or microwave until cheese melts. Finish off with an orange.

Afternoon snack: A crisp apple

Dinner: Roast pork with trimmings

Serve lean roast pork (about 4 oz) with ½ cup natural apple sauce, a medium-sized cooked sweet potato, 1 cup steamed zucchini, and green salad. Add a glass of wine if you like, and top the meal off with 8 ounces light vanilla or lemon yogurt sprinkled with ½ cup diced mango.

SATURDAY

GI:	47
Total Energy:	1690 cal
Fat:	50 g
Carbohydrate:	215 g
Fiber:	27 g

■

Breakfast: Egg, toast, and apple juice
One egg, prepared as desired (use vegetable spray if cooking in a pan). Toast two slices of pumpernickel bread and spread with 1 tablespoon of light margarine. Include 4-ounce glass of apple juice.

Morning snack: Four Social Tea biscuits with tea or coffee

Lunch: A healthy wrap
Wrap ½ cup tabouli, 2½-ounces veggie burger (crumbled), 1 cup shredded lettuce, one small tomato, and 1 ounce low-fat shredded cheese in a 2-ounce soft tortilla.

Afternoon snack: Two kiwis

Dinner: Pasta with mushroom and chicken marsala
Gently sauté 1 cup mushrooms with ½ cup scallions, garlic, fresh parsley, and 1–2 tablespoons of marsala wine. When the vegetables are cooked, toss in 3 ounces diced cooked chicken breast. Serve over 1½ cups steaming fettuccine. Accompany with 1 cup of sliced tomato and oregano salad mixed with fat-free Italian dressing.

Evening snack: Raisin Toast
One slice spread with 1 tablespoon light cream cheese.

SUNDAY

GI:	50
Total Energy:	1439 cal
Fat:	27 g
Carbohydrate:	204 g
Fiber:	25 g

■

Breakfast: Toast and hot chocolate

Spread two slices of 100% stoneground whole-wheat toast with 2 tablespoons part skim goat or cottage cheese. Serve with hot chocolate made with skim milk. Add one medium grapefruit.

Morning snack: A low fat granola bar

Lunch: Soup and salad

Heat up 1 cup tomato soup. Prepare a large tossed salad with mixed fresh vegetables and 2 ounces grilled chicken breast. Top with your favorite low-calorie-fat free dressing.

Afternoon snack: An ice cream cone

One scoop (½ cup) low fat ice cream.

Dinner: Fish, fries, and salad

Cut up 6 ounces of new potato into strips, spray with cooking oil, spread on baking tray, and bake in a very hot oven until browned. Wrap a piece of fresh fish (about 5 oz) in foil with fresh or dried herbs, lemon juice, and/or white wine. Bake it for the last 10–15 minutes with the potatoes. Toss together lettuce, cucumber and shallots with vinegar and 1 teaspoon olive oil.

Evening snack: A bunch of grapes or ¾ cup berries with a dollop of Cool Whip Lite

Did You Know?

YOU'RE LESS LIKELY to overeat if you eat high carbohydrate, low GI foods. They'll make you feel full (or even too full) and satisfied before you've eaten more than your body needs.

◀ 16 ▶

THE LOW-GI CHECKLIST

*G*OING GROCERY SHOPPING? Bring this list with you. It will help you choose low-GI foods quickly and easily.

BREADS

100% stoneground whole-wheat
100% stoneground whole-wheat pita
100% Whole-Grain, Natural Ovens
chapati (Baisen)
Happiness Raisin Pecan, Natural Ovens
Hearty 7 Grain, Healthy Choice
Hunger Filler, Natural Ovens
Multi-Grain Stay Trim, Natural Ovens
Natural Wheat, Natural Ovens
Nutty Natural, Natural Ovens
pumpernickel, whole-grain
rye

sourdough
sourdough rye
spelt, multigrain

BREAKFAST CEREALS

All-Bran, Kellogg's
apple and cinnamon hot cereal, ConAgra
Bran Buds with Psyllium™, Kellogg's
Bran Buds, Kellogg's
Multi-Bran Chex™, Kellogg's
Complete Bran flakes, Kellogg's
Just Right, Kellogg's
muesli, natural
muesli, toasted
oat bran
oat bran, raw
Raisin Bran, Kellogg's
rice bran
rolled or old-fashioned oats

COOKIES AND CAKES

Biscuits, Social Tea™
bread, banana
cake, chocolate, with chocolate frosting
cake, pound
cake, sponge
cake, vanilla
cookies, Arrowroot
cookies, Hearty Oatmeal, FIFTY50

cookies, oatmeal
cookies, oatmeal, sugar free, FIFTY50
cookies, shortbread
muffin, apple cinnamon, from mix*
wafers, vanilla, cremefilled, FIFTY50

DAIRY PRODUCTS AND ALTERNATIVES

custard, homemade
ice cream, regular
milk, low-fat, chocolate, with aspartame
milk, low-fat, chocolate, with sugar
milk, skim
milk, whole
mousse, butterscotch, low-fat, Nestlé
mousse, chocolate, low-fat, Nestlé
mousse, French vanilla, low-fat, Nestlé
mousse, hazelnut, low-fat, Nestlé
mousse, mango, low-fat, Nestlé
mousse, mixed berry, low-fat, Nestlé
mousse, strawberry, low-fat, Nestlé
pudding, instant, chocolate, made with milk
pudding, instant, vanilla, made with milk
soy milk, reduced-fat
soy milk, whole
yogurt, low-fat, fruit, with aspartame
yogurt, low-fat, fruit, with sugar
yogurt, non-fat, French vanilla, with sugar
yogurt, non-fat, strawberry, with sugar

*Foods containing fat in excess of American Heart Association guidelines. Use these only once in a while and in small amounts.

FRUIT AND FRUIT PRODUCTS

apple, fresh
apricot, fresh
banana, fresh
cantaloupe, fresh
cherries, fresh
grapefruit, fresh
grapes, fresh
kiwi, fresh
mango, fresh
orange, fresh
papaya, fresh
peach, canned in natural juice
peach, fresh
pear, canned in pear juice
pear, fresh
plum, fresh
prunes, pitted
strawberries, fresh
strawberry jam

GRAINS

barley, cracked
barley, pearled
buckwheat
buckwheat groats
bulgur
rice, basmati
rice, brown
rice, Uncle Ben's® Cajun Style
rice, Uncle Ben's® Long Grain and Wild

rice, Uncle Ben's® Converted, Original
rolled oats

JUICES

apple, with sugar or artificial sweetener
carrot, fresh
grapefruit, unsweetened
pineapple, unsweetened
tomato, canned, no added sugar

LEGUMES

beans, baked, canned
beans, butter, dried and cooked
beans, kidney, canned
beans, lima, baby, frozen
beans, mung, cooked
beans, navy, dried and cooked
beans, pinto, cooked
beans, soy, canned
chickpeas/garbanzo beans, canned
lentils, green, dried and cooked
lentils, red, dried and cooked
peas, black-eyed
peas, split, yellow, cooked

Note: Canned legumes have higher GI values than the boiled varieties because the temperatures and pressures used in the canning process increase the digestibility of the starch. But canned legumes are still an excellent low-fat, high-fiber, nutrient-rich low-GI choice!

NOODLES AND PASTA

capellini
fettuccine, egg
gluten-free noodles, cornstarch
instant noodles
linguine, thick, fresh, durum wheat, white, fresh
linguine, thin, fresh, durum wheat
macaroni, plain, cooked
mung bean, Lungkow beanthread
ravioli
rice, fresh, cooked
spaghetti, cooked 22 minutes
spaghetti, cooked 5 minutes
spaghetti, protein enriched, cooked 7 minutes
spaghetti, whole wheat
spirali, cooked, durum wheat
star pastina, cooked 5 minutes
tortellini
vermicelli

SNACK FOODS

apple cinnamon snack bar, ConAgra
sashews
chocolate bar, milk, Cadbury's
chocolate bar, milk, Dove®, Mars
chocolate bar, milk, Nestlé
chocolate bar, white, Milky Bar®
corn chips, plain, salted, Doritos™
M&M's®, peanut
nougat

Nutella® chocolate hazelnut spread
Peanut Butter & Chocolate Chip snack bar
peanuts
pecans
potato chips, plain, salted
Twix® Cookie Bar, caramel

SOUPS

lentil, canned
minestrone, canned, ready-to-serve
tomato, canned

STARCHY VEGETABLES

corn, canned, no salt added
corn, fresh
peas
potato, new, canned
potato, sweet
yam

VEGETABLES

artichokes
avocado
bok choy
broccoli
cabbage
carrots, peeled, cooked

cassava (yucca), cooked with salt
cauliflower
celery
cucumber
French beans (runner beans)
leafy greens
lettuce
pepper
squash

Low GI Substitutes

High-GI Food	Low-GI Alternative
Bread, whole wheat or white	Bread containing a lot of whole grains such as pumpernickel or 100% stoneground whole wheat
Processed breakfast cereal	Unrefined cereal such as old-fashioned oats.
Cookies and crackers	Cookies made with dried fruit and whole grains such as oats
Cakes and muffins	Look for those made with fruit, oats, whole grains
Tropical fruits	Temperate climate fruits such as berries, apples, peaches, pears, and nectarines
Potato	Use new potatoes, sweet potato, yam, or substitute with corn, peas, pasta, rice, or legumes
Rice	Try basmati, Uncle Ben's Original Converted™, brown, or long grain rice, or substitute with barley, noodles, or pasta

Making the Change

SOME PEOPLE CHANGE their diet easily, but for the majority of us, change of any kind is difficult. Changing our diet is seldom just a matter of giving up certain foods. A healthy diet contains a wide variety of foods but we need to eat them in appropriate proportions. If you are considering changes to your diet, keep these four guidelines in mind:

1. Aim to make changes gradually.
2. Attempt the easiest changes first.
3. Break big goals into a number of smaller, more achievable goals.
4. Accept lapses in your habits.
5. If you feel like you need some extra help, seek out some professional assistance from a dietitian.

◀ 17 ▶

YOUR QUESTIONS ANSWERED

Could a high-protein diet be harmful to a person with diabetes?

Yes. People with diabetes should avoid high-protein diets because eating large amounts of protein can tax the kidneys and bring on renal failure more quickly. (Renal failure is one possible complication of diabetes.) It's much healthier for people with diabetes to control their blood sugar by eating a low-GI diet.

What are the other side effects of a high-protein diet?

Some high-protein diets are also harmful for elderly people and anyone with high blood pressure or diabetes. High protein, high-fat diets can lead to high cholesterol, heart disease, and increase the risk of heart attack. These diets also lack fiber, which may lead to constipation. What's more, some high-protein diets can reduce the intake of important vitamins, minerals, fiber, and trace elements.

What's wrong with a low-carbohydrate diet?

There is little scientific evidence to back up or refute low-carbohydrate diets. One reason for the popularity of low-carbohydrate diets for weight loss is that initial loss is rapid. Within the first few days, the scales will be reading 4–7 pounds lower. That's a really encouraging sign to anyone trying to lose weight. The trouble is that most of that weight loss isn't body fat, but muscle glycogen and water.

When carbohydrate is no longer being supplied in sufficient amounts by your diet, the body uses its small carbohydrate reserves (muscle glycogen) to fuel muscle contraction. One gram of carbohydrate in the form of muscle and liver glycogen binds four grams of water. So when you use up your total reserves of 500 grams of glycogen within the first few days, you also lose 4 pounds of water, for a total loss of 5½ pounds, none of it fat. Conversely, when you return to normal eating, the carbohydrate reserves will be rapidly replenished along with the water, which is why there is an instant weight gain.

People who have followed low-carbohydrate diets for any length of time observe that the rate of weight loss plateaus off and they begin to feel rather tired and lethargic. That's not surprising because the muscles have little in the way of glycogen stores. Strenuous exercise requires both fat and carbohydrate in the fuel mix. So, long-term, these low-carbohydrate diets may discourage people from the physical exercise patterns that will help them keep their weight under control.

Our good advice is that the best diet for weight control is one you can stick to for life—one that includes your favorite foods and that accommodates your cultural and ethnic heritage and, prehaps most important, one that you can incorporate into your current lifestyle. This diet can vary somewhat in total carbohydrate, protein, and fat. At the present time, there is more scientific evidence supporting the use of bulky, higher carbohydrate, low-GI, low-fat diets for weight loss. But the bottom line is that the type of carbohydrate and the type of fat are critical. Choosing low-GI foods will not only promote weight control, it will reduce blood sugar levels after eating, increase satiety, and provide bulk and a rich supply of micronutrients.

Why are diets that disregard widely accepted nutritional guidelines so fashionable right now?

Several best-selling books have been published promoting high protein diets and generating a lot of publicity. But the fact is: Diets that limit major food groups do not work over the long haul.

A high-fat food may have a low glycemic index. Doesn't this give a falsely favorable impression of that food for people with diabetes?

Yes it does. The glycemic index of potato chips or French fries is lower than baked potatoes. The glycemic index of corn chips is lower than sweet corn. It is important not to base your food choices on the glycemic index alone; you need to consider the fat content and nutrient density of foods as well. Low-fat eating helps control weight, especially for people with diabetes.

Why should people with diabetes watch out for fatty foods?

With diabetes, being overweight and eating fatty foods prevents insulin from doing its job. When insulin can't work properly (or there isn't enough of it) blood sugar levels rise. Most type 2 diabetes is associated with an excess of abdominal fat (a "pot belly"). Breaded or battered foods, French fries, fried rice, pastries or other such fatty foods are often the cause of elevated blood sugar. The high glycemic index of potato, rice, or flour tends to increase blood sugar levels, and the extra fat interferes with the action of insulin and makes it less effective in clearing sugar from the blood.

Some foods high in fat have a low glycemic index and may seem all right to eat because of this. The glycemic index is low because fat tends to slow the rate of stomach emptying (and therefore the rate at which foods are digested in the small intestine). Some high fat foods, therefore, tend to have lower GI values than their low fat equivalents (potato chips, 54 compared with a dry baked potato, 85). This doesn't make them better foods.

If a food has a high glycemic index, should someone with diabetes avoid it?

Some foods like bread and potatoes have high GI values (70–80). But, potatoes and bread can play a major role in a high-carbohydrate and low-fat diet. You only have to exchange about half the carbohydrate (from high to low GI values) to achieve lower blood sugar levels. So, there's plenty of room for bread and potatoes. Some breads have lower GI values than others. Choose these if your goal is to lower the GI numbers as much as possible. You can't predict the GI value of a food from its composition. To test the GI number, you need real people and real foods. We describe how the GI value is measured on pages 30–31. Standardized methods are always followed so that results from one group of people can be directly compared with those from another.

Is it better to eat complex carbohydrate instead of simple sugars?

There are no big distinctions between sugars and starches in either nutritional terms or when it comes to GI values. Some sugars such as fructose (fruit sugar) have a low glycemic index. Others, such as glucose, have a high glycemic index. The most common sugar in our diet, ordinary table sugar (sucrose), has a moderate glycemic index.

Starches can fall into both the high and low GI categories too, depending on the type of starch and what treatment it has received during cooking and processing. Most modern starchy foods (such as bread, potatoes, and breakfast cereals), contain high- GI carbohydrate.

What our research has shown is that you don't have to eliminate sugar completely from your diet. However, it is important to remember that sugar alone won't keep the engine running smoothly, so don't overdo it. A balanced diet contains a wide variety of foods.

Are naturally occurring sugars better than refined sugars?

Naturally occurring sugars are those found in foods such as fruit, vegetables, and milk. Refined sugars are concentrated sources of sugar such as table sugar, honey, or molasses.

The rate of digestion and absorption of naturally occurring sugars is no different, on average, from that of refined sugars. There is wide variation within both food groups, depending on the food. For example, the glycemic index of fruits ranges from 22 for cherries to 72 for watermelon. Similarly, among the foods containing refined sugars, some have low GI values, while others have high GI numbers. The glycemic index of sweetened yogurt is only 33, while each Life Savers candy has a glycemic index of 70 (the same as some breads).

Some nutritionists argue that naturally occurring sugars are better because they contain minerals and vitamins not found in refined sugar. However, recent studies which have analyzed high sugar and low sugar diets clearly show that the diets overall contain similar amounts of micronutrients. Studies have shown that people who eat moderate amounts of refined sugars have perfectly adequate micronutrient intakes.

Can people with diabetes eat as much sugar as they want?

Research shows that moderate consumption of refined sugar (about 8 tsp a day) doesn't compromise blood sugar control. This means you can choose foods which contain refined sugar or even use small amounts of table sugar. Try to spread your sugar budget over a variety of nutrient-rich foods that sugar makes more palatable. Remember, sugar is concealed in many foods—a can of soft drink contains about 40 grams of sugar.

Most foods containing sugar do not raise blood sugar levels any more than most starchy foods. Golden Grahams (GI value of 71) contain 39 percent sugar while Rice Chex (GI value of 89) contain very little sugar. Many foods with large amounts of sugar have GI values close to 60—lower than white bread.

Sugar can be a source of enjoyment and help you limit your intake of high-fat foods, but the blood sugar response to a food is hard to predict. Use the tables in this book and your own blood sugar monitoring as a guide.

Some breads and potatoes have high GI values (70–80). Does this mean a person with diabetes should avoid all breads and potatoes?

Potatoes and bread can play a major role in a high carbohydrate and low fat diet, even if a secondary goal is to reduce the overall GI value. Only about half the carbohydrate has to be exchanged from high glycemic index to low glycemic index to achieve measurable improvements in diabetes control. So, there is still room for bread and potatoes. Of course, some types of bread and potatoes have lower GI values than others and these should be preferred if the goal is to lower the glycemic index as much as possible.

In the overall management of diabetes, the most

important message is that the diet should be low in fat and high in carbohydrate. This will help people not only to lose weight, but to keep it off and improve their overall blood glucose and lipid control.

◀ 18 ▶

GI SUCCESS STORIES

*J*UST IN CASE you're not yet convinced that a low-GI diet can help you manage your diabetes, dietitian Johanna Burani, M.S., R.D., C.D.E., offers these five real-life examples from her own practice. Many of Johanna's patients have controlled their diabetes, lost weight, and gained overall better health by choosing a low-GI way of life.

Margarine: Friend or Foe?

YOU'LL NOTICE THAT in some of the meals, Johanna suggests using light margarine. As you may know, many margarines are sources of trans fats, which can raise cholesterol levels and have been implicated in increased risk of heart attacks and possibly even breast cancer. Luckily, not all margarine is created equal! Some products now on store shelves clearly boast that they are trans-fat free (look for those). Here are some other guidelines Johanna suggests you follow to avoid these unhealthy fats:

■ Buy margarine by the tub, not the stick.
■ Look for "light," "low-fat," "non-fat" or "fat-free" on the label.
■ Make sure the first ingredient says "liquid," such as "liquid corn oil" or "liquid safflower oil."
■ Try a vegetable spread containing plant stanol esters.

CASE STUDY #1: GESTATIONAL DIABETES
"Marianne"

Age:	30
Height:	5'6"
Weight:	198 pounds, pre-pregnancy (clinically defined as "morbidly obese")

Background:

Married with a three-year-old daughter, Marianne is a stay-at-home mom. She doesn't smoke or drink alcohol, and for exercise she walks and plays with her daughter. During the third trimester of her last pregnancy, Marianne was diagnosed with pre-eclampsia (a toxemia accompanied by high blood pressure, water retention and protein in the urine). Her last child was born two weeks early by C-section.

This pregnancy, Marianne suffers from gestational diabetes, which was diagnosed in her seventh month of pregnancy. She takes no medications other than prenatal vitamins.

Marianne's "before" diet:
   Breakfast: 2 cups Team cereal, 4 ounces skim milk, 4 ounces orange juice
   Snack: 2 cups watermelon
   Lunch: Bowl of chicken noodle soup, six saltines, one piece of string cheese, butterscotch candy, 1 cup unsweetened canned peaches, water
   Snack: 2 cups watermelon
   Dinner: Large baked potato with sour cream, small baked chicken cutlet, sliced cucumber, water
   Late night snack: ½ bag popcorn, water

Marianne's "Before" Nutritional Analysis:

Calories:	1400
Carbohydrate:	237 g (70%)
Protein:	59 g (17%)
Fat:	19 g (13%)
GI:	73

Johanna's nutritional assessment:

Marianne is grossly underconsuming in all food categories except starches. Her caloric intake is meeting only about two thirds of her current needs. She should try to eliminate all processed foods high in sodium (such as canned soups) and should increase her dairy foods to at least 24 ounces of milk or the equivalent.

Along with increasing her milk intake, Marianne needs to increase her protein sources by adding 6 ounces of high quality proteins (poultry, fish, eggs, meats, and so on) pro-portioned throughout the day (three meals plus a bedtime snack). She also needs to increase her vegetable portions at both lunch and dinner, and include condiments to help provide the required 35 percent calories from fat.

GI-specific counseling:

Marianne should try to replace her current cereal and cracker choices with whole-grain options, substitute high-GI fruits (watermelon and pineapple) with low-GI options (apples, cherries, grapefruit, peaches, and so on) and replace the baked potato with noodles or long grain rice. Those changes will help produce lower-GI meals that will help regulate Marianne's blood sugar levels for the duration of her pregnancy.

Marianne's new, low-GI menu:

Breakfast: Two slices 100% stoneground whole-wheat toast, two pats butter, one egg, 8 ounces 2% milk

Snack: Small bran muffin, 8 ounces low-fat plain yogurt

Lunch: Roast beef (2 oz) sandwich with two slices sourdough bread, a tomato and cucumber salad dressed with 2 tablespoons salad dressing, 4 ounces unsweetened canned peaches, water

Snack: 1 ounce. potato chips, 4 ounces apple juice

Dinner: 1 cup spaghetti with marinara sauce, a 2-ounce meatball, 1 cup asparagus tips, 2 pats butter, medium orange, water

Snack: An 8-ounce glass of 2% milk, three graham cracker squares, and 1 tablespoon natural peanut butter (no added salt)

Marianne's "After" Nutritional Analysis:

Calories:	2100
Carbohydrate:	236 g (45%)
Protein:	101 g (19%)
Fat:	84 g (36%)
GI:	46

Marianne's winning results:

Marianne delivered a full-term healthy baby girl by C-section and gained a total of 17 pounds throughout her pregnancy. Her blood sugar remained within the normal ranges without the need of exogenous insulin, and her blood pressure was also stable and within normal ranges without medication.

Marianne's comments:

"I'm so relieved the pregnancy turned out so well. I was worried about the gestational diabetes, but we were able to control it with my diet. That's why I'm anxious to get on a permanent meal plan—it's the best way I can think of to prevent my getting type 2 diabetes."

CASE STUDY #2: TYPE 2 DIABETES
"Tony"

Age:	60
Height:	5'3"
Weight:	190 pounds

Background:

Tony is married, works as a full-time school administrator, and doesn't smoke or drink alcohol. For exercise, he walks for at least one hour every day. Tony has just been diagnosed with type 2 diabetes and was sent to Johanna to see whether dietary changes could control his diabetes so medication wouldn't be necessary. Tony also suffers from borderline high blood pressure.

Tony's "before" diet:

Breakfast: A small pastry or muffin, and coffee throughout the morning

Lunch: He usually skips lunch on work days; an occasional business lunch would consist of tuna steak, roll, cole slaw, French fries, and diet Coke

Dinner: Four hot dogs, tossed salad dressed with oil, vinegar, and bacon bits, small piece of Italian bread, diet iced tea and coffee

Snack: Glass of skim milk

> ## Tony's "Before" Nutritional Analysis:
>
> | | |
> |---|---|
> | Calories: | 2700 |
> | Carbohydrate: | 149 g (22%) |
> | Protein: | 154 g (23%) |
> | Fat: | 163 g (55%) |
> | GI: | 67 |

Johanna's nutritional assessment:

The best strategy to address Tony's multiple medical problems (diabetes, hypertension, obesity) all at once is to correct his diet. He would need to decrease his fat and sodium intake and increase his carbohydrates in the form of fruits, vegetables, and whole grains, and eat minimally processed foods. He should consume his daily calories in three meals and one or two snacks. He should attempt to drink 64 ounces of water throughout the day.

Tony needs to reduce his fat from his current 55 percent of calories to less than 30 percent. He needs to include three or four servings of fruit with meals and snacks. He needs to follow some brown bag lunch guidelines and identify the proper portion sizes for evening entrees, with an emphasis on low fat choices.

GI-specific counseling:

Although Tony's carbohydrate foods fall into the "intermediate GI" category, those foods contribute a paltry 22 percent of his caloric intake on an average day. His high-fat foods are making him feel full. He'll still feel full if he replaces these calorically dense foods with low-GI carbohydrates, but will be consuming less than half the calories.

Tony's new, low-GI menu:

 Breakfast: ¾ cup Raisin Bran, 8 ounces skim milk, coffee, ½ cup unsweetened canned peaches

 Lunch: Roasted turkey breast (2 oz) sandwich on two slices multigrain bread, 1 cup cantaloupe, water, or decaf diet beverage

 Snack: An 8-ounce container of light yogurt

 Dinner: One and a half cups fettuccine with marinara sauce, 3-ounce pan fried breaded pork cutlet, 1 tablespoon olive oil, 1 cup spinach, 4 ounces natural applesauce, water

 Snack: An 8-ounce cup of skim milk, oatmeal cookie

Tony's "After" Nutritional Analysis:

Calories:	1500
Carbohydrate:	211 g (55%)
Protein:	86 g (22%)
Fat:	39 g (23%)
GI:	43

Tony's winning results:

Tony reached his initial goal weight of 160 pounds after five months of eating low-GI meals and snacks. He takes no medications for either diabetes or high blood pressure. At my recommendation, he will maintain this weight for the next two to three months, at which time we'll design a new meal plan and exercise program to promote further gradual loss of another 10–20 pounds.

Tony's comments:

"I've never felt better in my life!"

CASE STUDY #3: TYPE 1 DIABETES
"Joyce"

Age:	64
Height:	5'6"
Weight:	227 pounds

pre-pregnancy (clinically
defined as "morbidly obese")

Background:

Joyce is an unmarried professional full-time cook. She
neither smokes nor drinks alcohol and walks every day
for 20 minutes (when she isn't feeling sick). Joyce has a
number of health problems: She suffers from high blood
pressure and is taking multiple medications to control
her diabetes. She also injects insulin twice a day (total of
111 units) and takes one oral agent as well. Her blood
sugar numbers range above 330, indicating poor control.
Joyce's cholesterol is also high, though she takes no medications for that condition.

Joyce's "before" diet:

Breakfast: Fried egg, two slices of whole-wheat toast
with margarine, coffee with 2% milk

Snack: An 8-ounce glass of apple juice

Lunch: Baked fish, ½ cup hash brown potatoes,
creamed spinach, apple, water

Dinner: Two slices of pizza, a handful of chips, two
bologna slices, apple, water

Late night snack: Handful of pretzel nuggets

Joyce's "Before" Nutritional Analysis:

Calories:	2200
Carbohydrate:	235 g (42%)
Protein:	87 g (15%)
Fat:	106 g (43%)
GI:	56

Johanna's nutritional assessment:

Because Joyce is morbidly obese and carries her excess fat abdominally, her body is resistant to insulin; even though she is taking large doses, her sugar control remained unsatisfactory. Joyce will need to reduce her caloric intake (specifically her fat calories) and balance her diet with more vegetables and low-fat dairy foods.

GI-specific counseling:

Joyce's carbohydrate choices consist predominantly of low- or intermediate-GI foods, which is a good start. By balancing her meals and snacks with more whole-grains, vegetables and low-fat dairy foods, and reducing her fat calories, she will start losing some weight and become less insulin-resistant, without feeling hungry. Her low-GI food choices will simultaneously help lower her weight, blood sugars, blood pressure, and cholesterol levels and give her more energy.

Joyce's new, low-GI menu:

Breakfast: 1⅓ cups of All-Bran with Extra Fiber, 8 ounces of skim milk, small apple

Lunch: 1 cup noodles, 4-ounce broiled chicken breast, 1 cup green beans, tossed salad dressed with 1 teaspoon olive oil and vinegar, 3 ounces cherries, water

Dinner: ⅔ cup Uncle Ben's Original Converted rice, 4-ounce lemon sole, 1 cup steamed broccoli and cauliflower florets, 1 tablespoon light margarine, 1 cup grapes, water

Snack: Eight graham cracker squares and 8 ounces light yogurt

---

Joyce's "After" Nutritional Analysis:

Calories:	1700
Carbohydrate:	224 g (53%)
Protein:	90 g (21%)
Fat:	47 g (26%)
GI:	43

Joyce's winning results:

In the past six years, Joyce has lost 47 pounds, and has been able to maintain a weight of 180. Her blood pressure and cholesterol levels have normalized. She is taking one insulin injection a day, having reduced her insulin requirement by 85 percent. Her blood sugars are all within the normal range.

Joyce's comments:

"It's so nice to have energy again. And I have more time on my hands now to work on my hobbies, since I go to the doctor less often."

CASE STUDY #4: TYPE 1 DIABETES
"Harry"

Age:	61
Height:	6'
Weight:	185 pounds

Background:

As he was moving up the ranks in the Coast Guard, Harry, a career officer, was diagnosed with type 1 diabetes and forced into early retirement. He is now president of a small, successful food compnay and travels extensively nationwide. He fits in a 2–3 mile jog most days of the week and sails for pleasure when he can. He has been wearing an insulin pump for five years.

Harry's "before" diet:

Waking: Three glucose tablets

Breakfast: 2 cups corn flakes, 1 cup blueberries, 1 cup 1% milk

Lunch: 1 pint chicken noodle soup (from supermarket), cup oyster crackers, two containers light yogurt, medium banana

Snack: Apple cinnamon snack bar

Snack: Four glucose tablets

Snack: ½ cup peanuts

Dinner: Four meatballs, three pieces Italian bread, ¼ cup raisins

Snack: Glass of skim milk

```
┌─────────────────────────────────────────────┐
│              Harry's "Before"                │
│          Nutritional Analysis:               │
│                                              │
│     Calories:              2700              │
│     Carbohydrate:    374 g (55%)             │
│     Protein:         139 g (21%)             │
│     Fat:              73 g (24%)             │
│     GI:                      71              │
└─────────────────────────────────────────────┘
```

Johanna's nutritional assessment:

Harry is a solid, lean, athletic man who has been living with diabetes for half his life. Because he is prone to low blood sugars (or so he thought), he frequently eats large amounts of carbs and/or glucose tablets to "stay ahead" of his low readings. A typical day includes five readings below 65 and at least four readings above 200 (some as high as 449). A typical week includes at least two hypoglycemic episodes. Harry's goal is to minimize his very low readings and try to eliminate his very high readings. He came for nutritional counseling with high hopes.

GI-specific counseling:

The first thing to address in Harry's diet is the amount of carbs he normally consumes, primarily as starches (corn flakes, white breads and crackers, snack bars) as well as the high-GI nature of these choices. Since he tests before and after all meals and snacks, whenever Harry sees a high number (more than 200) he increases his insulin to bring it down—sometimes too far. Then he corrects his "low" with pure glucose tablets, eventually eats more high-GI carbs, producing another high reading. And so his roller coaster ride takes his blood sugar levels up and down all day and night. By changing to low-GI foods, there will be a slower, steadier rise in his glucose levels, leaving him feeling more satisfied and energized. Measuring his glucose levels after low GI-meals and snacks, Harry will discover less of a need to correct highs with more insulin or lows with glucose tablets.

Harry's new, low-GI menu:

Breakfast: ½ cup old fashioned oats cooked in 1 cup 1% milk, 1 cup blueberries, 1 cup coffee

Snack: 1 cup light yogurt

Lunch: Large salad with various raw vegetables, 4 ounces. cheese, 1 cup fresh fruit salad, light yogurt, two to four small oatmeal cookies

Snack: Handful of peanuts

Dinner: Grilled chicken breast, 2 cups spaghetti with fresh tomato and basil sauce, 2 cups sauteed zucchini

Snack: Large baked apple, ½ cup light yogurt

Harry's "After" Nutritional Analysis:

Calories:	2200
Carbohydrate:	272 g (48%)
Protein:	125 g (22%)
Fat:	74 g (30%)
GI:	43

Harry's winning results:

The best news of all is that Harry's hypoglycemic episodes are down to about once a month—a decrease of

88 percent over the past year. Because his glucose levels are more regulated, he needs about 20 percent less insulin. His most recent HbA1c result measured 6.5, which is well within the target range the American Diabetes Association recommends. Maintaining his weight at 183 pounds, Harry looks and feels great!

Harry's comments:

"Eating this way has been a very easy adjustment for me. It has taken away the guilt, something that all people with diabetes feel. We all want to do the right thing. Eating low-GI foods is the right thing because these are the foods that help balance other choices. When I see healthy blood sugar levels, I feel good about myself. The glycemic index makes me feel like I'm in the fight!"

CASE STUDY #5: TYPE 2 DIABETES
"Jim"

Age:	49
Height:	5'4"
Weight:	285 pounds

Background:

Jim is a computer programmer and an avid outdoor photographer. Living alone, his 12-hour-plus workday leaves little time or energy to prepare a healthy evening meal or to think about breakfast or lunch food for the next day. Neither a drinker nor a smoker, Jim's only exercise is photographic walks on the weekends. He was diagnosed with type 2 diabetes at age 44, has high blood pressure, elevated cholesterol, and, with a BMI of 42, is clinically considered to be severely obese.

Jim's "before" diet:

Breakfast: Two eggs over easy, two thin slices of buttered white toast, 8 ounces. orange juice, three mugs black coffee throughout the morning.

Lunch: Commercially prepared frozen dinner, small green salad, 2 tablespoons ranch dressing

Dinner: Commercially prepared frozen dinner, 2 cups brussels sprouts, 1½ tablespoons tub margarine

(Throughout the course of the day, Jim also drank 4 liters of Diet Coke and admits that the food diary above represents a "very good day.")

Jim's "Before" Nutritional Analysis:

Calories:	Approximately 1500
Carbohydrate:	155 g (42%)
Protein:	81 g (22%)
Fat:	58 g (36%)
GI:	69

Johanna's nutritional assessment:

Jim knew he needed to improve his health. By focusing on weight-loss strategies, Jim agreed, his other health concerns would improve. He would need to increase his daily calories—especially fruits, vegetables and dairy foods. He should significantly reduce his caffeine intake

and choose water as his most-consumed beverage
throughout the day.

GI-specific counseling:

The big eye-catcher here is the amount of caffeine
Jim consumes between his coffee and Diet Cokes
(almost 5000 mg or neatly 9 times the amount nutritionists consider an acceptable daily intake). In such
high amounts, caffeine can have a hyperglycemic effect
on blood sugar levels. Although virtually calorie-free (he
deliberately chose *diet* soda and drank his coffee black),
Jim's beverages were putting him on a blood sugar roller
coaster, much as eating high-GI foods would. Because
he wanted to lose weight, as soon as he felt hungry, he
would just drink more caffeine. This quieted his hunger,
albeit for a short time. Jim actually was just setting him-
self up with a high blood sugar and then a crashing low.
He was spinning his wheels.

Jim's new, low-GI menu:

Breakfast: Two slices whole grain pumpernickel, one
   egg over easy, two clementines, water

Lunch: Two ounces whole-wheat pita, ½ cup tuna
   salad (store bought), handful cherry tomatoes,
   apple, water

Snack: 1 cup light fruited yogurt, two oatmeal cookies, water

Dinner: Commercially prepared frozen dinner (looked
   for lowest sodium and highest fiber options), 2 cups
   broccoli, apple, water

Snack: 4 ounces skim milk, apple cinnamon snack
   bar

(Jim decided to eliminate all diet soda and enjoys one 16-ounce mug of coffee throughout the morning.)

Jim's "After" Nutritional Analysis:

Calories:	1900
Carbohydrate:	250 g (54%)
Protein:	104 g (22%)
Fat:	50 g (24%)
GI:	44

Jim's winning results:

After eight months of revamping his diet, Jim has lost 55 pounds (BMI of 35). He is two thirds of the way to achieving his goal weight of 200 pounds. He no longer takes one of his two diabetes medications, and his HbA1c has come into the normal range (4.5). His last blood pressure check measured 110/70 and his lipid profile was almost completely normal. He is hoping his doctor will decrease or even eliminate his blood pressure and cholesterol medications as he approaches his goal weight.

Jim's comments:

"I never thought I could get through a day without lots of caffeine. I have so much more energy now that I've taken to climbing stairs during work hours."

19

LOW FAT, LOW-GI
RECIPE SECRETS

*A*s we have said constantly throughout this book, it is important to eat a high-carbohydrate and low-fat diet. The following practical tips that we have set out in an easy A to Z format will help you reduce the fat content of some of your favorite recipes while lowering their GI value.

KEY INGREDIENTS MAKE A BIG DIFFERENCE

Alcohol: Although excessive alcohol consumption can be fattening, as an ingredient in a recipe, alcohol itself won't create a high-calorie dish. Alcohol evaporates during cooking, so you lose most of the calories and are left with the flavor. A little wine in a sauce can give a delicious flavor, and sherry in an Asian-style marinade is essential.

Bacon: Bacon is a flavorful ingredient in many recipes because of the flavor it offers. You can make a little bacon go a long way by trimming off all fat and chopping it finely. Lean ham can be a more economical and leaner way to go. In casseroles and soups, a ham bone imparts a fine flavor without much fat.

Cheese: Several commonly used cheeses, such as American, Cheddar, and blue, contain more than 70 percent of their calories as fat. So cheese can be an ingredient that adds quite a bit of fat to a recipe. Although there are a number of fat-reduced cheeses available, many of these lose a lot in flavor for a small reduction in fat. It is worth comparing fat per ounce between brands to find the tastiest one with the lowest fat content. Alternatively, a sprinkle of a very tasty, grated cheese or Parmesan may do the job.

Part-skim ricotta and cottage cheeses are lower-fat alternatives to butter on a sandwich. It's worth trying some fresh part-skim ricotta from a deli—you may find the texture and flavor more acceptable than that of the ricotta available in containers in the supermarket. Flavored cottage cheeses are ideal low-fat toppings for crackers. Try part skim or light ricotta in lasagna instead of a creamy white sauce.

Cream and sour cream: Keep to very small amounts, as these are high in saturated fat. Substitute non-fat sour cream, which tastes very similar to the full-fat variety. A 16-ounce container of heavy cream can be poured into ice-cube trays and frozen, providing small servings of cream easily when you need it. Adding one ice-cube block (1 oz) of cream to a dish adds only 5½ grams of fat.

Dried beans, peas, and lentils: These legumes are all low in fat, high in fiber and protein, and very nutritious. Incorporating them in a recipe, perhaps as a partial substitution for meat, will lower the fat content of the finished product.

Eggs: Be conscious of eggs in a recipe, as they can add fat. Sometimes just the beaten egg white can be substituted for the whole egg, or use egg substitute.

Filo pastry: Unlike most other pastry, filo (also known as phyllo) is low in fat. To keep it that way, brush between the sheets with skim milk instead of melted butter when you prepare it. Look for it in the freezer section of the supermarket with other prepared pastry and use it as a strudel wrap.

Grilling: Grill or broil, rather than fry, tender cuts of meat, chicken and fish. Marinating first will add flavor, moisture, and tenderness.

Health food stores: Health food stores can be traps for the unwary. Check out the high-fat ingredients, such as hydrogenated vegetable oil, nuts, coconut, and palm kernel oil in products such as granola bars, fruit bars, and "healthy" cakes, (even if made with whole wheat-flour) that they stock on their shelves.

Ice cream: Ice cream is a source of carbohydrate, calcium, riboflavin, retinol, and protein. Low-fat varieties have the lower glycemic index—definitely a nutritious and tasty treat.

Jam: A tablespoon of jam on toast contains far fewer calories than a pat of butter.

Keep jars on hand: Bottled minced garlic, chili, or ginger can spice up your cooking in an instant.

Lemon juice: Try a fresh squeeze with ground black pepper on vegetables instead of a pat of butter. Lemon juice provides acidity that slows gastric emptying and lowers the GI value.

Milk: Many people dislike skim milk, particularly when they taste it on its own or in their coffee. However, you can use skim milk in a recipe and no one will notice— and the fat savings is great. For convenience you might want to keep powdered skim milk in the pantry, which can be made up to the desired quantity when you need it. It will taste more like fresh milk if you mix the powder and water according to directions and refrigerate the milk overnight before using it. Ultrapasteurized milk is handy in the cupboard, too.

Nuts: Nuts are valuable for their vitamin E content, but they are also high in fat. To keep the fat content of a recipe low, the quantity of nuts should be small.

Oil: Most of our recipes call for no more than two teaspoons of oil. Any polyunsaturated or monounsaturated oil is suitable. Cooking spray or brushing oil lightly over the base of the pan is ideal. If you find the amount of oil insufficient, cover your pan, or add a few drops of water and use steam to cook the ingredients without burning. It is a good idea to invest in a nonstick frying pan if you don't have one.

Pasta: Pasta is a food to eat more of and a great source of carbohydrate and B vitamins. Fresh or dried, the preparation is easy. Just boil in water until tender or "al dente," drain, and top with a dollop of pesto, grilled or steamed vegetables, tomato sauce, or a sprinkle of Parmesan and pepper. Pasta may appear in your menu as a side dish to meat, as noodles in soup, as a meal in itself with chicken or shrimp or vegetables, or even as an ingredient in a dessert.

Questions: Ask your dietitian for more recipe ideas. (See "For More Information" on page 169 to locate an R.D. near you.)

Reduce: Lower the fat content of ground beef by browning it in a nonstick pan, then placing the meat in a colander and pouring boiling water through it to wash away the fat. Return to the pan to continue cooking. It is a good idea to buy the better-quality (90% to 93% lean) ground beef with less fat.

Stock: If you are prepared to go to the effort of making your own stock—good for you! Prepare it in advance, refrigerate it, then skim off the accumulated fat from the top. Prepared stock is available in long-life cartons and cans in the supermarket. Stock cubes are another alternative. Look for brands that have reduced salt.

Sauté: Heat the pan first, brush with the recommended amount of oil (or less), add the food and cook, stirring lightly over gentle heat.

Use spices: Underlying the need for fat is a need for taste. Be creative with other flavorings.

Vinegar: A vinaigrette dressing (1 tablespoon vinegar and 2 tablespoons of oil) with your salad can lower the blood-sugar response to the whole meal by up to 30 percent. The best types of vinegars for this purpose are red and white wine vinegars. You can also use lemon juice.

Weighing: What's the weight of the meat you're buying? Start noticing the weight that appears on the butcher's scales or package label and consider how many servings it will give you. With a food such as steak, which is basically all edible meat, 3–5 ounces per serving is sufficient. One pound is enough for four portions. Choose lean cuts of meat and trim away the fat before cooking or before you put it away. Alternate meat or chicken with fish once or twice a week.

Yogurt: Yogurt is a valuable food in many ways. It is a good source of calcium, "friendly bacteria," protein, and riboflavin, and, unlike milk, is suitable for people who are lactose intolerant. Low-fat plain yogurt is a suitable substitute for sour cream. If you're using yogurt in a hot sauce or casserole, add it at the last minute and do not let it boil, or it will curdle. It is best if you can bring the yogurt to room temperature before adding it to the hot dish. To do this, mix a small amount of yogurt with a little sauce from the dish, then stir this mixture back into the bulk of the sauce.

Zero fat: Eating zero fat is unhealthy, so speak with a dietitian about how to get just the right amount you need. Our bodies need essential fatty acids that can't be synthesized and must be supplied in the diet. Fat does add flavor—use it to your advantage.

◀ 20 ▶

LET'S TALK GLYCEMIC LOAD

*I*N ADDITION TO the GI values we provide in this book, our tables also include the glycemic load (GL) value for average-sized food portions. Taken together, the glycemic index and glycemic load provide you with all the information you need to choose a diet brimming with health-boosting foods.

GLYCEMIC LOAD 101

A food's glycemic load results from the GI value and carbohydrate per serving of food. When we eat a carbohydrate-containing meal, our blood glucose first rises, then falls. The extent to which it rises and remains high is critically important to our health and depends on two things: the *amount* of a carbohydrate in the meal and the *nature* (GI value) of that carbohydrate. Both factors equally determine blood-glucose changes.

Researchers at Harvard University came up with a way of combining and describing these two factors with the term "glycemic load," which not only provides a measure of the level of glucose in the blood, but also the insulin demand produced by a normal serving of the food. Researchers measure GI values for fixed portions of foods containing a certain amount of carbohydrate (usually 50). Then, as people eat different-sized portions of the same foods, we can work out the extent to which a certain portion of food will raise the blood-glucose level by calculating a glycemic load value for that amount of food.

To calculate glycemic load, multiply a food's GI value by the amount of carbohydrate in a particular serving size, then divide by 100.

■

**Glycemic load =
(GI x carbohydrate per serving) ÷ 100**

■

For example, a small apple has a GI value of 40 and contains 15 grams of carbohydrate. Its glycemic load is (40 × 15) ÷ 100 = 6. A small 5-ounce potato has a GI value of 90 and 15 grams of carbohydrate. It has a glycemic load of (90 × 15) ÷ 100 = 14. This means one small potato will raise your blood-glucose level higher than one apple.

■

**Low GL = 10 or less
Intermediate GL = 11–19
High GL = 20 or more**

■

How GI Values Affect
Glycemic Load

THE GLYCEMIC LOAD is greatest for those foods that provide the highest-GI carbohydrate, particularly those we tend to eat in large quantities. Compare the glycemic load of the following foods to see how the serving size, as well as the GI value, help to determine the glycemic response:

Rice, 1 cup	Spaghetti, 1 cup
Carbohydrates: 43	Carbohydrates: 40
GI: 83	GI: 44
GL: 36	GL: 18
$(83 \times 43) \div 100 = 36$	$(44 \times 40) \div 100 = 18$

Some nutritionists argue that the glycemic load is an improvement on the glycemic index because it provides an estimate of both quantity *and* quality of carbohydrate (the GI value gives us just quality) in a diet. In large Harvard studies, however, researchers were able to predict disease risk from people's overall diet, as well as its glycemic load. Using the glycemic load strengthened the relationship, suggesting that the more frequently we consume high-carbohydrate, high-GI foods, the worse it is for our health. Carbohydrate by itself has no effect—in other words, there was no benefit of low carbohydrate intake over high carbohydrate intake, or vice versa.

If you make the mistake of using GL alone, you might find yourself eating a diet with very little carbohydrate but a lot of fat and excessive amounts of protein. That's why you need to use the glycemic index to compare foods of similar nature (such as bread with bread) and use the glycemic load when you're deciding on the portion size of the carbohydrates you want to eat. If you use the technique correctly, GL values will guide you to eat smaller portions of high GI foods.

Remember that the GL values we provide are for the standardized (nominal) portion sizes listed. If you eat a different portion size, then you'll need to calculate another GI value. Here's how: First, determine the size of your portion, then work out the available carbohydrate content of this weight (this value is listed next to the GL), then multiply by the food's GI value. For example, the nominal serving size listed for bran flakes is $\frac{1}{2}$ cup, the available carbohydrate is 18 grams, and the GI value is 74. So the GL for a $\frac{1}{2}$-cup serving of bran flakes is $(74 \times 18) \div 100 = 13$. If, however, you normally eat 1 cup of bran flakes, you'd need to double the available carbohydrate $(18 \times 2 = 36)$ and the GL for your larger cereal portion would be $(74 \times 36) \div 100 = 27$. These numbers show that the larger portion of cereal releases a larger quantity of glucose into the bloodstream.

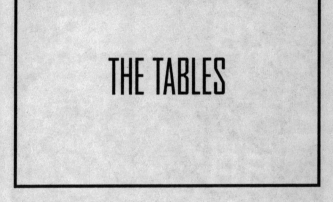

THE TABLES

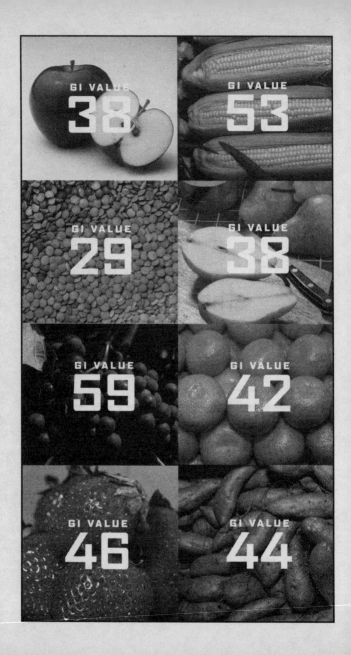

GI VALUE
38

GI VALUE
53

GI VALUE
29

GI VALUE
38

GI VALUE
59

GI VALUE
42

GI VALUE
46

GI VALUE
44

◆ 21 ◆

A TO Z GI VALUES

THE TABLE IN this section will help you find a food's glycemic index value quickly and easily, because we've listed the foods alphabetically.

The list provides not only the food's GI value but also its glycemic load (GL = (carbohydrate content × GI) ÷ 100). We calculate the glycemic load using a nominal, or standardized, serving size as well as the carbohydrate content of that serving—both of which we've also listed. That way, you can choose foods with either a low GI value or a low glycemic load. If your favorite food is both high-GI and high-GL, you can either cut down the serving size or dilute the GL by combining it with very low-GI foods, such as rice and lentils.

For the first time, we've also included foods that have very little carbohydrate; their GI value is zero, indicated by [0]. Many vegetables, such as avocados and broccoli, and protein foods such as chicken, cheese, and tuna, fall into the low- or no-carbohydrate category. Most alcoholic beverages are also low in carbohydrate.

Key to the Table

GI: The glycemic index value for the food, where glucose equals 100

Nominal Serving Size: The portion of food tested

Net Carb per Serving: The total grams of carbs available to the body for digestion from the particular food in the specific serving size (total grams of carbs minus grams of fiber)

GL per Serving: Glycemic load of the food; this relates to the quantity of carbs that will enter the bloodstream for the particular food in the specific serving size

---

FOOD	GI Value	Nominal Serving Size	Net Carb per Serving	GL per Serving
A				
All-Bran®, breakfast cereal	30	½ cup	15	4
Almonds	[0]	1.75 oz	0	0
Angel food cake, 1 slice	67	¹⁄₁₂ cake	29	19
Apple, dried	29	9 rings	34	10
Apple, fresh, medium	38	4 oz	15	6
Apple juice, pure, unsweetened, reconstituted	40	8 oz	29	12
Apple muffin, small	44	3.5 oz	41	18
Apricots, canned in light syrup	64	4 halves	19	12
Apricots, dried	30	17 halves	27	8
Apricots, fresh, 3 medium	57	4 oz	9	5
Arborio, risotto rice, cooked	69	¾ cup	53	36
Artichokes (Jerusalem)	[0]	½ cup	0	0
Avocado	[0]	¼	0	0
B				
Bagel, white	72	½	35	25
Baked beans	38	⅔ cup	31	12
Baked beans, canned in tomato sauce	48	⅔ cup	15	7
Banana cake, 1 slice	47	⅛ cake	38	18
Banana, fresh, medium	52	4 oz	24	12
Barley, pearled, cooked	25	1 cup	42	11
Basmati rice, white, cooked	58	1 cup	38	22
Beef	[0]	4 oz	0	0
Beer	[0]	8 oz	10	0
Beets, canned	64	½ cup	7	5
Bengal gram dahl, chickpea	11	5 oz	36	4
Black bean soup	64	1 cup	27	17
Black beans, cooked	30	⅘ cup	23	7
Black-eyed peas, canned	42	⅔ cup	17	7

[0] indicates that the food has so little carbohydrate that the GI value cannot be tested. The GL, therefore, is 0.

FOOD	GI Value	Nominal Serving Size	Net Carb per Serving	GL per Serving
Blueberry muffin, small	59	3.5 oz	47	28
Bok choy, raw	[0]	1 cup	0	0
Bran Flakes™, breakfast cereal	74	½ cup	18	13
Bran muffin, small	60	3.5 oz	41	25
Brandy	[0]	1 oz	0	0
Brazil nuts	[0]	1.75 oz	0	0
Breton wheat crackers	67	6 crackers	14	10
Broad beans	79	½ cup	11	9
Broccoli, raw	[0]	1 cup	0	0
Broken rice, white, cooked	86	1 cup	43	37
Brown rice, cooked	50	1 cup	33	16
Buckwheat	54	¾ cup	30	16
Bulgur, cooked 20 min	48	¾ cup	26	12
Bun, hamburger	61	1.5 oz	22	13
Butter beans, canned	31	⅔ cup	20	6
C				
Cabbage, raw	[0]	1 cup	0	0
Cactus Nectar, Organic Agave, light, 90% fructose (Western Commerce)	11	1 Tbsp	8	1
Cactus Nectar, Organic Agave, light, 97% fructose (Western Commerce)	10	1 Tbsp	8	1
Cantaloupe, fresh	65	4 oz	6	4
Cappellini pasta, cooked	45	1½ cups	45	20
Carrot juice, fresh	43	8 oz	23	10
Carrots, peeled, cooked	49	½ cup	5	2
Carrots, raw	47	1 medium	6	3
Cashew nuts, salted	22	1.75 oz	13	3
Cauliflower, raw	[0]	¾ cup	0	0
Celery, raw	[0]	2 stalks	0	0
Cheese	[0]	4 oz	0	0

[0] indicates that the food has so little carbohydrate that the GI value cannot be tested. The GL, therefore, is 0.

FOOD	GI Value	Nominal Serving Size	Net Carb per Serving	GL per Serving
Cherries, fresh	22	18	12	3
Chicken nuggets, frozen	46	4 oz	16	7
Chickpeas, canned	42	⅔ cup	22	9
Chickpeas, dried, cooked	28	⅔ cup	30	8
Chocolate cake made from mix with chocolate frosting	38	4 oz	52	20
Chocolate milk, low-fat	34	8 oz	26	9
Chocolate mousse, 2% fat	31	½ cup	22	7
Chocolate powder, dissolved in water	55	8 oz	16	9
Chocolate pudding, made from powder and whole milk	47	½ cup	24	11
Choice DM™, nutritional support product, vanilla (Mead Johnson)	23	8 oz	24	6
Clif® bar (cookies & cream)	101	2.4 oz	34	34
Coca Cola®, soft drink	53	8 oz	26	14
Cocoa Puffs™, breakfast cereal	77	1 cup	26	20
Complete™, breakfast cereal	48	1 cup	21	10
Condensed milk, sweetened	61	2½ Tbsps	27	17
Converted rice, long-grain, cooked 20–30 min, Uncle Ben's®	50	1 cup	36	18
Converted rice, white, cooked 20–30 min, Uncle Ben's®	38	1 cup	36	14
Corn Flakes™, breakfast cereal	92	1 cup	26	24
Corn Flakes™, Honey Crunch, breakfast cereal	72	¾ cup	25	18
Corn pasta, gluten-free	78	1¼ cups	42	32
Corn Pops™, breakfast cereal	80	1 cup	26	21
Corn Thins, puffed corn cakes, gluten-free	87	1 oz	20	18
Corn, sweet, cooked	60	½ cup	18	11
Cornmeal, cooked 2 min	68	1 cup	13	9
Couscous, cooked 5 min	65	¾ cup	35	23

[0] indicates that the food has so little carbohydrate that the GI value cannot be tested. The GL, therefore, is 0.

FOOD	GI Value	Nominal Serving Size	Net Carb per Serving	GL per Serving
Cranberry juice cocktail	52	8 oz	31	16
Crispix™, breakfast cereal	87	1 cup	25	22
Croissant, medium	67	2 oz	26	17
Cucumber, raw	[0]	¾ cup	0	0
Cupcake, strawberry-iced, small	73	1.5 oz	26	19
Custard apple, raw, flesh only	54	4 oz	19	10
Custard, homemade	43	½ cup	26	11
Custard, prepared from powder with whole milk, instant	35	½ cup	26	9
D				
Dates, dried	50	7	40	20
Desiree potato, peeled, cooked	101	5 oz	17	17
Doughnut, cake type	76	1.75 oz	23	17
E				
Eggs, large	[0]	2	0	0
Enercal Plus™ (Wyeth-Ayerst)	61	8 oz	40	24
English Muffin™ bread (Natural Ovens)	77	1 oz	14	11
Ensure™, vanilla drink	48	8 oz	34	16
Ensure™ bar, chocolate fudge brownie	43	1.4 oz	20	8
Ensure Plus™, vanilla drink	40	8 oz	47	19
Ensure Pudding™, old-fashioned vanilla	36	4 oz	26	9
F				
Fanta®, orange soft drink	68	8 oz	34	23
Fettuccine, egg, cooked	32	1½ cups	46	15
Figs, dried	61	3	26	16
Fish	[0]	4 oz	0	0
Fish sticks	38	3.5 oz	19	7
Flan/crème caramel	65	½ cup	73	47
French baguette, white, plain	95	1 oz	15	15

[0] indicates that the food has so little carbohydrate that the GI value cannot be tested. The GL, therefore, is 0.

FOOD	GI Value	Nominal Serving Size	Net Carb per Serving	GL per Serving
French fries, frozen, reheated in microwave	75	30 pcs	29	22
French green beans, cooked	[0]	½ cup	0	0
French vanilla cake made from mix, with vanilla frosting	42	4 oz	58	24
French vanilla ice cream, premium, 16% fat	38	½ cup	14	5
Froot Loops™, breakfast cereal	69	1 cup	26	18
Frosted Flakes™, breakfast cereal	55	1 cup	26	15
Fructose, pure	19	1 Tbsp	10	2
Fruit cocktail, canned, light syrup	55	½ cup	16	9
Fruit leather	61	2 pcs	24	15
G				
Gatorade™ (orange) sports drink	89	8 oz	15	13
Gin	[0]	1 oz	0	0
Glucerna™, vanilla (Abbott)	31	8 oz	23	7
Glucose (dextrose)	99	1 Tbsp	10	10
Glucose tablets	102	3 pcs	15	15
Gluten-free corn pasta	78	1½ cups	42	32
Gluten-free multigrain bread	79	1 oz	13	10
Gluten-free rice and corn pasta	76	1½ cups	49	37
Gluten-free spaghetti, rice and split pea, canned in tomato sauce	68	8 oz	27	19
Gluten-free split pea and soy pasta shells	29	1½ cups	31	9
Gluten-free white bread, sliced	80	1 oz	15	12
Glutinous (sticky) rice, white, cooked	92	⅔ cup	48	44
Gnocchi	68	6 oz	48	33
Grapefruit, fresh, medium	25	1 half	11	3
Grapefruit juice, unsweetened	48	8 oz	20	9
Grape-Nuts® (Post), breakfast cereal	75	¼ cup	21	16

[0] indicates that the food has so little carbohydrate that the GI value cannot be tested. The GL, therefore, is 0.

FOOD	GI Value	Nominal Serving Size	Net Carb per Serving	GL per Serving
Grapes, black, fresh	59	¾ cup	18	11
Grapes, green, fresh	46	¾ cup	18	8
Green peas	48	⅓ cup	7	3
Green pea soup, canned	66	8 oz	41	27
H				
Hamburger bun	61	1.5 oz	22	13
Happiness™ (cinnamon, raisin, pecan bread) (Natural Ovens)	63	1 oz	14	9
Hazelnuts	[0]	1.75 oz	0	0
Healthy Choice™ Hearty 100% Whole Grain	62	1 oz	14	9
Healthy Choice™ Hearty 7 Grain	55	1 oz	14	8
Hearty Oatmeal cookies, FIFTY50	30	4 cookies	20	6
Honey	55	1 Tbsp	18	10
Hot cereal, apple & cinnamon, dry (ConAgra)	37	1.2 oz	22	8
Hot cereal, unflavored, dry (ConAgra)	25	1.2 oz	19	5
Hunger Filler™, whole-grain bread (Natural Ovens)	59	1 oz	13	7
I				
Ice cream, low-fat, vanilla, "light"	50	½ cup	9	5
Ice cream, premium, French vanilla, 16% fat	38	½ cup	14	5
Ice cream, premium, "ultra chocolate," 15% fat	37	½ cup	14	5
Ice cream, regular fat	61	½ cup	20	12
Instant potato, mashed	97	¾ cup	20	17
Instant rice, white, cooked 6 min	74	¾ cup	42	36
Ironman PR® bar, chocolate	39	2.3 oz	26	10

[0] indicates that the food has so little carbohydrate that the GI value cannot be tested. The GL, therefore, is 0.

FOOD	GI Value	Nominal Serving Size	Net Carb per Serving	GL per Serving
J				
Jam, apricot fruit spread, reduced sugar	55	1½ Tbsps	13	7
Jam, strawberry	51	1½ Tbsps	20	10
Jasmine rice, white, cooked	109	1 cup	42	46
Jelly beans	78	10 large	28	22
K				
Kaiser roll	73	1 half	16	12
Kavli™ Norwegian crispbread	71	5 pcs	16	12
Kidney beans, canned	52	⅔ cup	17	9
Kidney beans, cooked	23	⅔ cup	25	6
Kiwi fruit	53	4 oz	12	7
Kudos® Whole Grain Bars, chocolate chip	62	1.8 oz	32	20
L				
Lactose, pure	46	1 Tbsp	10	5
Lamb	[0]	4 oz	0	0
Leafy vegetables (spinach, arugula, etc.), raw	[0]	1½ cups	0	0
L.E.A.N Fibergy™ bar, Harvest Oat	45	1.75 oz	29	13
L.E.A.N Life long Nutribar™, Chocolate Crunch	32	1.5 oz	19	6
L.E.A.N Life long Nutribar™, Peanut Crunch	30	1.5 oz	19	6
L.E.A.N Nutrimeal™, drink powder, Dutch Chocolate	26	8 oz	13	3
Lemonade, reconstituted	66	8 oz	20	13
Lentil soup, canned	44	9 oz	21	9
Lentils, brown, cooked	29	¾ cup	18	5
Lentils, green, cooked	30	¾ cup	17	5
Lentils, red, cooked	26	¾ cup	18	5

[0] indicates that the food has so little carbohydrate that the GI value cannot be tested. The GL, therefore, is 0.

FOOD	GI Value	Nominal Serving Size	Net Carb per Serving	GL per Serving
Lettuce	[0]	4 leaves	0	0
Life Savers®, peppermint candy	70	18 pcs	30	21
Light rye bread	68	1 oz	14	10
Lima beans, baby, frozen	32	¾ cup	30	10
Linguine pasta, thick, cooked	46	1½ cups	48	22
Linguine pasta, thin, cooked	52	1½ cups	45	23
Liquor	[0]	1.5 oz	0	0
Long-grain rice, cooked 10 min	61	1 cup	36	22
Lychees, canned in syrup, drained	79	4 oz	20	16

M

FOOD	GI Value	Nominal Serving Size	Net Carb per Serving	GL per Serving
M & M's®, peanut	33	15 pcs	17	6
Macadamia nuts	[0]	1.75 oz	0	0
Macaroni and cheese, made from mix	64	1 cup	51	32
Macaroni, cooked	47	1¼ cups	48	23
Maltose	105	1 Tbsp	10	11
Mango	51	4 oz	15	8
Maple syrup, pure Canadian	54	1 Tbsp	18	10
Marmalade, orange	48	1½ Tbsps	20	9
Mars Bar®	68	2 oz	40	27
Melba toast, Old London	70	6 pcs	23	16
METRx® bar (vanilla)	74	3.6 oz	50	37
Milk Arrowroot™ cookies	69	5	18	12
Millet, cooked	71	⅔ cup	36	25
Mini Wheats™, whole-wheat breakfast cereal	58	12 pcs	21	12
Mousse, butterscotch, 1.9% fat	36	1.75 oz	10	4
Mousse, chocolate, 2% fat	31	1.75 oz	11	3
Mousse, hazelnut, 2.4% fat	36	1.75 oz	10	4
Mousse, mango, 1.8% fat	33	1.75 oz	11	4
Mousse, mixed berry, 2.2% fat	36	1.75 oz	10	4

[0] indicates that the food has so little carbohydrate that the GI value cannot be tested. The GL, therefore, is 0.

FOOD	GI Value	Nominal Serving Size	Net Carb per Serving	GL per Serving
Mousse, strawberry, 2.3% fat	32	1.75 oz	10	3
Muesli bar containing dried fruit	61	1 oz	21	13
Muesli bread, made from mix in bread oven (ConAgra)	54	1 oz	12	7
Muesli, gluten-free, with low-fat milk	39	1 oz	19	7
Muesli, Swiss Formula	56	1 oz	16	9
Muesli, toasted	43	1 oz	17	7
Multi-Grain 9-Grain bread	43	1 oz	14	6

N

FOOD	GI Value	Nominal Serving Size	Net Carb per Serving	GL per Serving
Navy beans, canned	38	5 oz	31	12
Nesquik™, chocolate dissolved in low-fat milk, no-sugar-added	41	8 oz	11	5
Nesquik™, strawberry dissolved in low-fat milk, no-sugar-added	35	8 oz	12	4
New creamer potato, canned	65	5 oz	18	12
New creamer potato, unpeeled and cooked 20 min	78	5 oz	21	16
Noodles, instant "two-minute" (Maggi®)	46	1½ cups	40	19
Noodles, mung bean (Lungkow beanthread), dried, cooked	39	1½ cups	45	18
Noodles, rice, fresh, cooked	40	1½ cups	39	15
Nutella®, chocolate hazelnut spread	33	1 Tbsp	12	4
Nutrigrain™, breakfast cereal	66	1 cup	15	10
Nutty Natural™, whole-grain bread (Natural Ovens)	59	1 oz	12	7

O

FOOD	GI Value	Nominal Serving Size	Net Carb per Serving	GL per Serving
Oat bran, raw	55	2 Tbsp	5	3
Oatmeal, cooked 1 min	66	1 cup	26	17
Oatmeal cookies	55	4 small	21	12
Oatmeal cookies, Sugar-Free, FIFTY50	47	4 cookies	28	10

[0] indicates that the food has so little carbohydrate that the GI value cannot be tested. The GL, therefore, is 0.

FOOD	GI Value	Nominal Serving Size	Net Carb per Serving	GL per Serving
Orange juice, unsweetened, reconstituted	53	8 oz	18	9
Orange, fresh, medium	42	4 oz	11	5
P				
Pancakes, buckwheat, gluten-free, made from mix	102	2 4" pancakes	22	22
Pancakes, made from mix	67	2 4" pancakes	58	39
Papaya, fresh	59	4 oz	8	5
Parsnips	97	½ cup	12	12
Pastry	59	2 oz	26	15
Pea soup, canned	66	8 oz	41	27
Peach, canned in heavy syrup	58	½ cup	26	15
Peach, canned in light syrup	52	½ cup	18	9
Peach, fresh, large	42	4 oz	11	5
Peanuts	14	1.75 oz	6	1
Pear halves, canned in natural juice	43	½ cup	13	5
Pear, fresh	38	4 oz	11	4
Peas, green, frozen, cooked	48	½ cup	7	3
Pecans	[0]	1.75 oz	0	0
Pepper, fresh, green or red	[0]	3 oz	0	0
Pineapple, fresh	66	4 oz	10	6
Pineapple juice, unsweetened	46	8 oz	34	15
Pinto beans, canned	45	⅔ cup	22	10
Pinto beans, dried, cooked	39	¾ cup	26	10
Pita bread, white	57	1 oz	17	10
Pizza, cheese	60	1 slice	27	16
Pizza, Super Supreme, pan (11.4% fat)	36	1 slice	24	9
Pizza, Super Supreme, thin and crispy (13.2% fat)	30	1 slice	22	7
Plums, fresh	39	2 medium	12	5
Pop Tarts™, double chocolate	70	1.8 oz pastry	36	25

[0] indicates that the food has so little carbohydrate that the GI value cannot be tested. The GL, therefore, is 0.

FOOD	GI Value	Nominal Serving Size	Net Carb per Serving	GL per Serving
Popcorn, plain, cooked in microwave oven	72	1½ cups	11	8
Pork	[0]	4 oz	0	0
Potato chips, plain, salted	54	2 oz	21	11
Potato, baked	85	5 oz	30	26
Potato, microwaved	82	5 oz	33	27
Pound cake (Sara Lee)	54	2 oz	28	15
PowerBar® (chocolate)	57	2.3 oz	42	24
Premium soda crackers	74	5 crackers	17	12
Pretzels	83	1 oz	20	16
Prunes, pitted	29	6	33	10
Pudding, instant, chocolate, made with whole milk	47	½ cup	24	11
Pudding, instant, vanilla, made with whole milk	40	½ cup	24	10
Puffed crispbread	81	1 oz	19	15
Puffed rice cakes, white	82	3 cakes	21	17
Puffed Wheat, breakfast cereal	80	2 cups	21	17
Pumpernickel rye kernel bread	41	1 oz	12	5
Pumpkin	75	3 oz	4	3

R

FOOD	GI Value	Nominal Serving Size	Net Carb per Serving	GL per Serving
Raisin Bran™, breakfast cereal	61	½ cup	19	12
Raisins	64	½ cup	44	28
Ravioli, meat-filled, cooked	39	6.5 oz	38	15
Red wine	[0]	3.5 oz	0	0
Red-skinned potato, peeled and microwaved on high for 6–7.5 min	79	5 oz	18	14
Red-skinned potato, peeled, boiled 35 min	88	5 oz	18	16
Red-skinned potato, peeled, mashed	91	5 oz	20	18

[0] indicates that the food has so little carbohydrate that the GI value cannot be tested. The GL, therefore, is 0.

FOOD	GI Value	Nominal Serving Size	Net Carb per Serving	GL per Serving
Resource Diabetic™, nutritional support product, vanilla (Novartis)	34	8 oz	23	8
Rice and corn pasta, gluten-free	76	1½ cups	49	37
Rice bran, extruded	19	1 oz	14	3
Rice cakes, white	78	3 cakes	21	17
Rice Krispies™, breakfast cereal	82	1¼ cups	26	22
Rice Krispies Treat™ bar	63	1 oz	24	15
Rice noodles, fresh, cooked	40	1½ cups	39	15
Rice, parboiled	72	1 cup	36	26
Rice pasta, brown, cooked 16 min	92	1½ cups	38	35
Rice vermicelli	58	1½ cups	39	22
Rolled oats	42	1 cup	21	9
Roll-Ups®, processed fruit snack	99	1 oz	25	24
Roman (cranberry) beans, fresh, cooked	46	¾ cup	18	8
Russet, baked potato	85	5 oz	30	26
Rutabaga, fresh, cooked	72	5 oz	10	7
Rye bread	58	1 oz	14	8
Ryvita® crackers	69	3 crackers	16	11
S				
Salami	[0]	4 oz	0	0
Salmon	[0]	4 oz	0	0
Sausages, fried	28	3.5 oz	3	1
Scones, plain	92	1 oz	9	8
Sebago potato, peeled, cooked	87	5 oz	17	14
Seeded rye bread	55	1 oz	13	7
Semolina, cooked (dry)	55	⅓ cup	50	28
Shellfish (shrimp, crab, lobster, etc.)	[0]	4 oz	0	0
Sherry	[0]	2 oz	0	0
Shortbread cookies	64	1 oz	16	10
Shredded Wheat™, breakfast cereal	75	⅔ cup	20	15

[0] indicates that the food has so little carbohydrate that the GI value cannot be tested. The GL, therefore, is 0.

FOOD	GI Value	Nominal Serving Size	Net Carb per Serving	GL per Serving
Shredded Wheat™ biscuits	62	1 oz	18	11
Skim milk	32	8 oz	13	4
Skittles®	70	45 pcs	45	32
Smacks™, breakfast cereal	71	¾ cup	23	11
Smoothie, raspberry (ConAgra)	33	8 oz	41	14
Snack bar, Apple Cinnamon (ConAgra)	40	1.75 oz	29	12
Snack bar, Peanut Butter & Choc-Chip (ConAgra)	37	1.75 oz	27	10
Snickers® bar	68	2.2 oz	35	23
Social Tea Biscuits	55	6 cookies	19	10
Soda crackers, Premium	74	5 crackers	17	12
Soft drink, Coca Cola®	53	8 oz	26	14
Soft drink, Fanta®, orange	68	8 oz	34	23
Sourdough rye	48	1 oz	12	6
Sourdough wheat	54	1 oz	14	8
Soy & Flaxseed bread (mix in bread oven) (ConAgra)	50	1 oz	10	5
Soybeans, canned	14	1 cup	6	1
Soybeans, dried, cooked	20	1 cup	6	1
Spaghetti, durum wheat, cooked 20 min	64	1½ cups	43	27
Spaghetti, gluten-free, rice and split pea, canned in tomato sauce	68	8 oz	27	19
Spaghetti, white, cooked 5 min	38	1½ cups	48	18
Spaghetti, whole wheat, cooked 5 min	32	1½ cups	44	14
Special K™, breakfast cereal	69	1 cup	21	14
Spirali pasta, durum wheat, al dente	43	1½ cups	44	19
Split pea and soy pasta shells, gluten-free	29	1½ cups	31	9
Split pea soup	60	1 cup	27	16
Split peas, yellow, cooked 20 min	32	¾ cup	19	6
Sponge cake, plain	46	2 oz	36	17

[0] indicates that the food has so little carbohydrate that the GI value cannot be tested. The GL, therefore, is 0.

FOOD	GI Value	Nominal Serving Size	Net Carb per Serving	GL per Serving
Squash, raw	[0]	⅔ cup	0	0
Star pastina, white, cooked 5 min	38	1½ cups	48	18
Stay Trim™, whole-grain bread (Natural Ovens)	70	1 oz	15	10
Stoned Wheat Thins	67	14 crackers	17	12
100% stone-ground whole-wheat bread	53	1 slice	13	7
Strawberries, fresh	40	4 oz	3	1
Strawberry jam	51	1½ Tbsps	20	10
Strawberry shortcake	42	2.2 oz	40	17
Stuffing, bread	74	1 oz	21	16
Sucrose	68	1 Tbsp	10	7
Super Supreme pizza, pan (11.4% fat)	36	1 slice	24	9
Super Supreme pizza, thin and crispy (13.2% fat)	30	1 slice	22	7
Sushi, salmon	48	3.5 oz	36	17
Sweet corn, whole kernel, canned, diet-pack, drained	46	1 cup	28	13
Sweet potato, cooked	44	5 oz	25	11
T				
Taco shells, baked	68	2 shells	12	8
Tapioca, cooked with milk	81	¾ cup	18	14
Tofu-based frozen dessert, chocolate with high-fructose (24%) corn syrup	115	1.75 oz	9	10
Tomato juice, canned, no added sugar	38	8 oz	9	4
Tomato soup	38	1 cup	17	6
Tortellini, cheese	50	6.5 oz	21	10
Tortilla chips, plain, salted	63	1.75 oz	26	17
Total™, breakfast cereal	76	¾ cup	22	17
Tuna	[0]	4 oz	0	0
Twix® Cookie Bar, caramel	44	2 cookies	39	17

[0] indicates that the food has so little carbohydrate that the GI value cannot be tested. The GL, therefore, is 0.

FOOD	GI Value	Nominal Serving Size	Net Carb per Serving	GL per Serving
U				
Ultra chocolate ice cream, premium, 15% fat	37	½ cup	14	5
Ultracal™ with fiber (Mead Johnson)	40	8 oz	29	12
V				
Vanilla cake made from mix, with vanilla frosting	42	4 oz	58	24
Vanilla pudding, instant, made with whole milk	40	½ cup	24	10
Vanilla wafers, creme-filled, FIFTY50	41	4 cookies	20	8
Vanilla wafers	77	6 cookies	18	14
Veal	[0]	4 oz	0	0
Vermicelli, white, cooked	35	1½ cups	44	16
W				
Waffles, Aunt Jemima®	76	1 4" waffle	13	10
Walnuts	[0]	1.75 oz	0	0
Water crackers	78	7 crackers	18	14
Watermelon, fresh	72	4 oz	6	4
Weet-Bix™, breakfast cereal	69	2 biscuits	17	12
Wheaties™, breakfast cereal	82	1 cup	21	17
Whiskey	[0]	1 oz	0	0
White bread	70	1 oz	14	10
White rice, instant, cooked 6 min	87	1 cup	42	36
Wine (red or white)	[0]	5 oz	0	0
100% Whole Grain™ bread (Natural Ovens)	51	1 oz	13	7
Whole milk	31	8 oz	12	4
Whole-wheat bread	77	1 oz	12	9
Wonder™ white bread	80	1 oz	14	11

[0] indicates that the food has so little carbohydrate that the GI value cannot be tested. The GL, therefore, is 0.

FOOD	GI Value	Nominal Serving Size	Net Carb per Serving	GL per Serving
X				
Xylitol	8	1 Tbsp	10	1
Y				
Yam, peeled, cooked	37	5 oz	36	13
Yogurt, low-fat, wild strawberry	31	8 oz	34	11
Yogurt, low-fat, with fruit and artificial sweetener	14	8 oz	15	2
Yogurt, low-fat, with fruit and sugar	33	8 oz	35	12

[0] indicates that the food has so little carbohydrate that the GI value cannot be tested. The GL, therefore, is 0.

◆ 22 ◆

LOW TO HIGH GI VALUES

FOR THOSE WHO wish to choose a diet with the lowest GI values possible, we've created the following listing in order of GI values (i.e., from lowest to highest value). We've also divided the list into food categories, so that when you want to find a low-GI vegetable or fruit, for example, the information is at your fingertips. The categories are:

- bakery products
- beverages
- breads
- breakfast foods
- cookies
- crackers
- dairy products and alternatives
- fruits and fruit products
- grains
- infant formulas and baby foods

- legumes
- meal-replacement products
- mixed meals and convenience foods
- noodles
- pasta
- protein foods
- snack foods and candy
- soups
- special dietary products
- sugars
- vegetables

As we discuss in *The New Glucose Revolution*, it's not necessary to eat all of your carbohydrates from low-GI sources. If half of your carbohydrate choices have low GI values, you're doing well. If you also eat a low-GI food at each meal, you'll be reducing the GI values overall.

FOOD	LOW	INTERMEDIATE	HIGH

BAKERY PRODUCTS

Cakes

FOOD	LOW	INTERMEDIATE	HIGH
Banana	○		
Chocolate, with chocolate frosting	○		
Pound	○		
Sponge	○		
Vanilla	○		
Angel food		◑	
Flan		◑	

Muffins

FOOD	LOW	INTERMEDIATE	HIGH
Apple with sugar or artificial sweeteners	○		
Apple, oat, and raisin	○		
Banana, oat, and honey		◑	
Bran		◑	
Blueberry		◑	
Carrot		◑	
Oatmeal, made from mix, Quaker Oats™		◑	
Cupcake, iced			●
Scone, plain			●

Pastries

FOOD	LOW	INTERMEDIATE	HIGH
Croissant		◑	
Doughnut, cake-type			●

BEVERAGES

Alcoholic

FOOD	LOW	INTERMEDIATE	HIGH
Beer	○		

FOOD	LOW	INTERMEDIATE	HIGH
Brandy	○		
Gin	○		
Sherry	○		
Whiskey	○		
Wine, red	○		
Wine, white	○		
Juices			
Apple, with sugar or artificial sweetener	○		
Carrot, fresh	○		
Grapefruit, unsweetened	○		
Pineapple, unsweetened	○		
Tomato, canned, no added sugar	○		
Smoothies and Shakes			
Raspberry	○		
Soy	○		
Soft drinks			
Coca-Cola®		◐	
Fanta®		◐	
Sports drinks			
Gatorade®			●

BREADS

FOOD	LOW	INTERMEDIATE	HIGH
Fruit			
Muesli, made from mix	○		
Natural Ovens Happiness™, cinnamon, raisin, pecan		◐	
Gluten-free			
Fiber-enriched			●
White			●

FOOD	LOW	INTERMEDIATE	HIGH
Rye			
Pumpernickel	○		
Sourdough	○		
Cocktail		◑	
Light		◑	
Whole wheat		◑	
Spelt			
Multigrain	○		
White			●
Wheat			
100% stone-ground whole-wheat bread	○		
100% Whole Grain	○		
Soy & Linseed bread machine mix	○		
Flatbread, Indian		◑	
Hearty 7 Grain		◑	
Pita, plain		◑	
Bagel			●
Baguette			●
Bread stuffing			●
English Muffin			●
Flatbread, Middle Eastern			●
Italian			●
Lebanese, white			●
White, enriched			●
Whole wheat			●

FOOD	LOW	INTERMEDIATE	HIGH

BREAKFAST FOODS

Breakfast cereal bars

FOOD	LOW	INTERMEDIATE	HIGH
Rice Krispies® Treat		◐	

Cooked cereals

FOOD	LOW	INTERMEDIATE	HIGH
Hot cereal, apple & cinnamon, ConAgra	○		
Old-fashioned oats	○		
Cream of Wheat™, regular, Nabisco		◐	
One Minute Oats, Quaker Oats		◐	
Quick Oats, Quaker Oats		◐	
Cream of Wheat™, instant, Nabisco			●
Oatmeal, instant			●

Grain products

FOOD	LOW	INTERMEDIATE	HIGH
Pancakes, prepared from mix	○		
Pancakes, buckwheat, gluten-free, made from mix			●
Waffles, Aunt Jemima®			●

Ready-to-eat cereals

FOOD	LOW	INTERMEDIATE	HIGH
All-Bran®, Kellogg's	○		
Complete™ Bran Flakes, Kellogg's	○		
Bran Buds™, Kellogg's		◐	
Bran Chex™, Kellogg's		◐	
Froot Loops™, Kellogg's		◐	
Frosted Flakes™, Kellogg's		◐	
Just Right™, Kellogg's		◐	
Life™, Quaker Oats		◐	
Nutrigrain™, Kellogg's		◐	
Oat bran, raw, Quaker Oats		◐	
Puffed Wheat, Quaker Oats		◐	

FOOD	LOW	INTERMEDIATE	HIGH
Raisin Bran™, Kellogg's		◑	
Special K™, Kellogg's		◑	
Bran Flakes™, Kellogg's			●
Cheerios™, General Mills			●
Corn Chex™, Kellogg's			●
Corn Flakes™, Kellogg's			●
Corn Pops™, Kellogg's			●
Grapenuts™, Post			●
Rice Krispies™, Kellogg's			●
Shredded Wheat™, Nabisco			●
Team™ Flakes, Nabisco			●
Total™			●
Weetabix™			●

COOKIES

FOOD	LOW	INTERMEDIATE	HIGH
Hearty Oatmeal, FIFTY50	○		
Oatmeal, Sugar-Free, FIFTY50	○		
Social Tea Biscuits	○		
Vanilla wafers, creme filled, FIFTY50	○		
Arrowroot		◑	
Digestives		◑	
Tea biscuits		◑	
Shortbread		◑	
Vanilla wafers			●

CRACKERS

FOOD	LOW	INTERMEDIATE	HIGH
Breton wheat		◑	
Melba toast		◑	
Rye crispbread		◑	
Ryvita™		◑	
Stoned Wheat Thins		◑	

FOOD	LOW	INTERMEDIATE	HIGH
Water		◑	
Kavli™ Norwegian Crispbread			●
Premium soda (Saltines)			●
Rice cakes, puffed			●

DAIRY PRODUCTS AND ALTERNATIVES

Custard

	LOW	INTERMEDIATE	HIGH
Homemade	○		

Ice cream

	LOW	INTERMEDIATE	HIGH
Regular	○		

Milk

	LOW	INTERMEDIATE	HIGH
Low-fat, chocolate, with aspartame	○		
Low-fat, chocolate, with sugar	○		
Skim	○		
Whole	○		
Condensed, sweetened			●

Mousse

	LOW	INTERMEDIATE	HIGH
Butterscotch, low-fat, Nestlé	○		
Chocolate, low-fat, Nestlé	○		
French vanilla, low-fat, Nestlé	○		
Hazelnut, low-fat, Nestlé	○		
Mango, low-fat, Nestlé	○		
Mixed berry, low-fat, Nestlé	○		
Strawberry, low-fat, Nestlé	○		

Pudding

	LOW	INTERMEDIATE	HIGH
Instant, chocolate, made with milk	○		
Instant, vanilla, made with milk	○		

FOOD	LOW	INTERMEDIATE	HIGH
Soy milk			
Reduced fat	O		
Whole	O		
Soy yogurt			
Tofu-based frozen dessert, chocolate			●
Yogurt			
Low-fat, fruit, with aspartame	O		
Low-fat, fruit, with sugar	O		
Nonfat, French vanilla, with sugar	O		
Nonfat, strawberry, with sugar	O		

FRUIT AND FRUIT PRODUCTS

FOOD	LOW	INTERMEDIATE	HIGH
Apple, fresh	O		
Apricot, fresh	O		
Banana, fresh	O		
Cantaloupe, fresh	O		
Cherries, fresh	O		
Grapefruit, fresh	O		
Grapes, fresh	O		
Mango, fresh	O		
Orange, fresh	O		
Peach, canned in natural juice	O		
Peach, fresh	O		
Pear, canned in pear juice	O		
Pear, fresh	O		
Plum, fresh	O		
Prunes, pitted	O		
Strawberries, fresh	O		
Strawberry jam	O		
Figs, dried		◑	
Fruit cocktail, canned		◑	

FOOD	LOW	INTERMEDIATE	HIGH
Kiwi, fresh	◑		
Papaya, fresh		◑	
Peach, canned in heavy syrup		◑	
Peach, canned in light syrup		◑	
Pineapple, fresh		◑	
Raisins/sultanas		◑	
Dates, dried			●
Lychee, canned in syrup, drained			●
Watermelon, fresh			●

GRAINS

FOOD	LOW	INTERMEDIATE	HIGH
Barley, cracked	○		
Barley, pearled	○		
Buckwheat	○		
Buckwheat groats	○		
Bulgur	○		
Corn, canned, no salt added	○		
Rice, brown	○		
Rice, Cajun Style, Uncle Ben's®	○		
Rice, Long Grain and Wild, Uncle Ben's®	○		
Rice, parboiled, converted, white, cooked 20–30 min, Uncle Ben's®	○		
Barley, rolled		◑	
Corn, fresh		◑	
Cornmeal		◑	
Couscous		◑	
Rice, arborio (risotto)		◑	
Rice, Basmati		◑	
Rice, Garden Style, Uncle Ben's®		◑	
Rice, parboiled, long grain, cooked 10 minutes		◑	

FOOD	LOW	INTERMEDIATE	HIGH
Millet			●
Rice, sticky			●
Rice, parboiled			●
Tapioca boiled with milk			●

INFANT FORMULA AND BABY FOODS

Baby foods

FOOD	LOW	INTERMEDIATE	HIGH
Apple, apricot, and banana, baby cereal		◐	
Chicken and noodles with vegetables, strained		◐	
Corn and rice, baby		◐	
Oatmeal, creamed, baby		◐	
Rice pudding, baby		◐	

Infant formula

FOOD	LOW	INTERMEDIATE	HIGH
SMA, 20 cal/fl oz, Wyeth	○		
Nursoy, soy-based, milk-free, Wyeth		◐	

LEGUMES

Beans

FOOD	LOW	INTERMEDIATE	HIGH
Baked, canned	○		
Butter, dried and cooked	○		
Kidney, canned	○		
Lima, baby, frozen	○		
Mung, cooked	○		
Navy, dried and cooked	○		
Pinto, cooked	○		
Soy, canned	○		

Lentils

FOOD	LOW	INTERMEDIATE	HIGH
Green, dried and cooked	○		
Red, dried and cooked	○		

FOOD	LOW	INTERMEDIATE	HIGH
Peas			
Black-eyed	○		
Chickpeas/garbanzo beans, canned	○		
Split, yellow, cooked	○		

MEAL-REPLACEMENT PRODUCTS

FOOD	LOW	INTERMEDIATE	HIGH
Designer chocolate, sugar free, Worldwide Sport Nutrition low carbohydrate products	○		
L.E.A.N Fibergy™ bar, Harvest Oat, Usana	○		
L.E.A.N (Life long) Nutribar™, Peanut Crunch, Usana	○		
L.E.A.N (Life long) Nutribar™, Chocolate Crunch, Usana	○		

MIXED MEALS AND CONVENIENCE FOODS

FOOD	LOW	INTERMEDIATE	HIGH
Chicken nuggets, frozen, reheated	○		
Fish fillet, reduced fat, breaded	○		
Fish sticks	○		
Greek lentil stew with a bread roll, homemade	○		
Lean Cuisine™, chicken with rice	○		
Pizza, Super Supreme, pan, Pizza Hut	○		
Pizza, Super Supreme, thin and crispy, Pizza Hut	○		
Pizza, Vegetarian Supreme, thin and crispy, Pizza Hut	○		
Spaghetti Bolognese	○		
Sushi, salmon	○		
Tortellini, cheese, Stouffer	○		
Tuna patty, reduced fat	○		
Cheese sandwich, white bread		◑	
Kugel		◑	
Macaroni and cheese, boxed, Kraft		◑	
Peanut-butter sandwich, white/whole-wheat bread		◑	
Pizza, cheese, Pillsbury		◑	

FOOD	LOW	INTERMEDIATE	HIGH
Spaghetti, gluten-free, canned in tomato sauce		◐	
Sushi, roasted sea algae, vinegar and rice		◐	
Taco shells, cornmeal-based, baked, El Paso		◐	
White bread and butter		◐	
Stir-fried vegetables with chicken and rice, homemade			●

NOODLES

FOOD	LOW	INTERMEDIATE	HIGH
Instant	○		
Mung bean, Lungkow beanthread	○		
Rice, fresh, cooked	○		
Rice, dried, cooked		◐	
Udon, plain, reheated 5 min		◐	

PASTA

FOOD	LOW	INTERMEDIATE	HIGH
Capellini	○		
Fettuccine, egg	○		
Gluten-free, cornstarch	○		
Linguine, thick, fresh, durum wheat, white	○		
Linguine, thin, fresh, durum wheat	○		
Macaroni, plain, cooked	○		
Ravioli	○		
Spaghetti, cooked 5 min	○		
Spaghetti, cooked 22 min	○		
Spaghetti, protein enriched, cooked 7 min	○		
Spaghetti, whole wheat	○		
Spirali, cooked, durum wheat	○		
Star pastina, cooked 5 min	○		
Tortellini	○		
Vermicelli	○		
Gnocchi		◐	

FOOD	LOW	INTERMEDIATE	HIGH
Rice vermicelli		◑	
Spaghetti, cooked 10 min, Barilla		◑	
Corn, gluten-free			●
Rice and corn, gluten-free			●
Rice, brown, cooked 16 min			●

PROTEIN FOODS

FOOD	LOW	INTERMEDIATE	HIGH
Beef	○		
Cheese	○		
Cold cuts	○		
Eggs	○		
Fish	○		
Lamb	○		
Pork	○		
Sausages	○		
Shellfish (shrimp, crab, lobster, etc.)	○		
Veal	○		

SNACK FOODS AND CANDY

Candy

FOOD	LOW	INTERMEDIATE	HIGH
Nougat	○		
Jelly beans			●
Life Savers®			●
Skittles®			●

Chips

FOOD	LOW	INTERMEDIATE	HIGH
Corn, plain, salted, Doritos™	○		
Potato, plain, salted	○		

Chocolate bars

FOOD	LOW	INTERMEDIATE	HIGH
Milk, Cadbury's	○		

FOOD	LOW	INTERMEDIATE	HIGH
Milk, Dove®, Mars	◯		
Milk, Nestlé	◯		
White, Milky Bar®	◯		
Mars Bar®		◑	
Snickers Bar®		◑	

Chocolate candy

M & M's®, peanut	◯		

Chocolate spread

Nutella®, chocolate hazelnut spread	◯		

Dried-fruit bars

Fruit Roll-Ups®			●

Nuts

Cashews	◯		
Peanuts	◯		
Pecans	◯		

Popcorn

Plain, microwaved			●

Pretzels

Plain, salted			●

Snack bars

Apple Cinnamon, ConAgra	◯		
Peanut Butter & Choc-Chip	◯		
Twix® Cookie Bar, caramel	◯		
Kudos Whole Grain Bars, chocolate chip		◑	

Sports bars

Ironman PR bar®, chocolate	◯		

FOOD	LOW	INTERMEDIATE	HIGH
PowerBar®, chocolate		◐	

SOUPS

	LOW	INTERMEDIATE	HIGH
Lentil, canned	○		
Minestrone, canned, ready-to-serve	○		
Tomato, canned	○		
Black bean, canned		◐	
Green pea, canned		◐	
Split pea, canned		◐	

SPECIAL DIETARY PRODUCTS

	LOW	INTERMEDIATE	HIGH
Choice DM™, vanilla, Mead Johnson	○		
Ensure™, Abbott	○		
Ensure Plus™, vanilla, Abbott	○		
Ensure Pudding™, vanilla, Abbott	○		
Ensure™ bar, chocolate fudge brownie, Abbott	○		
Ensure™, vanilla, Abbott	○		
Glucerna™ bar, lemon crunch, Abbott	○		
Glucerna™ SR shake, vanilla, Abbott	○		
Glucerna™, vanilla, Abbott	○		
Resource Diabetic™, vanilla, Novartis	○		
Resource Plus, chocolate, Novartis	○		
Ultracal™ with fiber, Mead Johnson	○		
Enercal Plus™, Wyeth-Ayerst		◐	
Enrich Plus shake, vanilla, Ross		◐	

SUGARS

	LOW	INTERMEDIATE	HIGH
Blue Agave, Organic Agave Cactus Nectar, light, 90% fructose, Western Commerce	○		
Blue Agave, Organic Agave Cactus Nectar, light, 97% fructose, Western Commerce	○		

FOOD	LOW	INTERMEDIATE	HIGH
Fructose	○		
Lactose	○		
Honey		◑	
Sucrose		◑	
Glucose			●
Maltose			●

VEGETABLES

FOOD	LOW	INTERMEDIATE	HIGH
Artichokes	○		
Avocado	○		
Bok choy	○		
Broccoli	○		
Cabbage	○		
Carrots, peeled, cooked	○		
Cassava (yucca), cooked with salt	○		
Cauliflower	○		
Celery	○		
Corn, canned, no salt added	○		
Cucumber	○		
French beans (runner beans)	○		
Leafy greens	○		
Lettuce	○		
Peas, frozen, cooked	○		
Pepper	○		
Potato, sweet	○		
Squash	○		
Yam	○		
Beet		◑	
Corn, sweet, cooked		◑	
Potato, boiled/canned		◑	
Potato, new, canned		◑	

FOOD	LOW	INTERMEDIATE	HIGH
Taro		◑	
Broad beans			●
Parsnips			●
Potato, French fries, frozen and reheated			●
Potato, instant			●
Potato, mashed			●
Potato, microwaved			●
Potato, russet, baked			●
Pumpkin			●
Rutabaga			●

FOR MORE INFORMATION

To find a dietitian
  The American Dietetic Association
  120 South Riverside Plaza
  Suite 2000
  Chicago, IL 60606
  Phone: 1-800-877-1600
  www.eatright.org

To order Natural Ovens bread
  Natural Ovens Bakery
  PO Box 730
  Manitowoc, WI 54221-0730
  Phone: 1-800-772 0730
  www.naturalovens.com

To order FIFTY50 Foods or find your nearest retailer:
  FIFTY50 Foods

PO Box 89
Mendham, NJ 07945
Phone: 1-973-543-7006
www.fifty50.com

Primary Care Physicians

If you think you need help with a weight problem, it's always a good idea to see your primary care physician for an evaluation.

Community Support Groups

Many communities offer support groups targeting people who are trying to lose weight. Your primary care physician or local hospital may be able to direct you to a support group best suited to your needs.

Diabetes Organizations

Extra weight can often make a diabetic condition worse. For more information about living with and controlling your diabetes, contact the following:

The American Diabetes Association
1701 North Beauregard Street
Alexandria, VA 22311
Phone: 1-800-DIABETES (1-800-342-2383)
www.diabetes.org

Canadian Diabetes Association
National Office
15 Toronto Street, Suite 800
Toronto, ON M5C 2E3
Phone: 1-416-363-3373
1-800-BANTING (1-800-226-8464)
www.diabetes.ca

GLYCEMIC INDEX TESTING

*I*F YOU ARE a food manufacturer, you may be interested in having the glycemic index value of some of your products tested on a fee-for-service basis. For more information, contact:

Sydney University Glycaemic Index Research Service
(SUGiRS)
Department of Biochemistry
University of Sydney
NSW 2006 Australia
Fax: (61) (2) 9351-6022
E-mail: j.brandmiller@mmb.usyd.edu.au

ACKNOWLEDGMENTS

*W*E WOULD LIKE to thank Linda Rao, M.Ed., for her editorial work on the American edition.

ABOUT THE AUTHORS

JENNIE BRAND-MILLER, PH.D., is Professor of Human Nutrition in the Human Nutrition Unit, School of Molecular and Microbial Biosciences at the University of Sydney, and President of the Nutrition Society of Australia. She has taught postgraduate students of nutrition and dietetics at the University of Sydney for over twenty-four years and currently leads a team of twelve research scientists, whose interests focus on all aspects of carbohydrate—diet and diabetes, the glycemic index of foods, insulin resistance, lactose intolerance, and oligosaccharides in infant nutrition. She has published sixteen books and 140 journal articles and is the co-author of all books in the *Glucose Revolution* series.

•

KAYE FOSTER-POWELL, M. NUTR. & DIET., is an accredited practicing dietitian with extensive experience in diabetes management. She has conducted research into the glycemic index of foods and its practical applications over the last fifteen years. Currently she is a dietitian with Wentworth Area Diabetes Services in New South Wales and consults on all aspects of the glycemic index. She is the co-author of all books in the *Glucose Revolution* series.

■

JOHANNA BURANI, M.S., R.D., C.D.E., is a Registered Dietitian and Certified Diabetes Educator with more than thirteen years' experience in nutritional counseling. The co-author of *The Glucose Revolution Life Plan* and principal author of *Good Carbs, Bad Carbs*, as well as several other books and professional manuals, she specializes in designing individual meal plans based on low-GI food choices. She lives in Mendham, New Jersey.

■

STEPHEN COLAGIURI, M.D., is the Director of the Diabetes Centre and Head of the Department of Endocrinology, Metabolism and Diabetes at the Prince of Wales Hospital in Randwick, New South Wales. He graduated from the University of Sydney in 1970 and received his Fellowship of the Royal Australasian College of Physicians in 1977. He has a joint academic appointment at the University of New South Wales. He has more than 100 scientific papers to his name, many concerned with the importance of carbohydrates in the diet of people with diabetes, and is the co-author of most books in the *Glucose Revolution* series.

Also Available

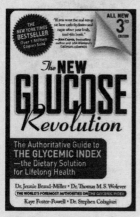

ISBN 978-1-56924-258-2 • $16.95

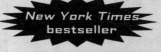

THE NEW GLUCOSE REVOLUTION, 3rd EDITON

Written by the world's foremost authorities on the subject, whose findings are supported by hundreds of studies from Harvard University's School of Public Health and other leading research centers, *The New Glucose Revolution* shows how and why eating low-GI foods has major health benefits for everybody seeking to establish a way of eating for lifelong health.

THE LOW GI DIET REVOLUTION

The only science-based diet proven to help you lose up to 10 percent of your current weight and develop a lifetime of healthy eating habits that can protect you from illness and disease. *The Low GI Diet Revolution* shows you how to make low-GI food choices for every meal that will satisfy your hunger, increase your energy levels, and eliminate your desire to eat more than you should.

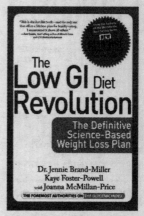

ISBN 978-1-56924-413-5 • $15.95

THE NEW GLUCOSE REVOLUTION LOW GI VEGETARIAN COOKBOOK

The perfect cookbook for vegetarians and vegans looking to eat the right carbs—and everyone seeking delicious recipes low on the glycemic index. Featuring beautiful color photos throughout and more than 80 creative, inspiring recipes, the book also includes information on the best nutrient sources and menu ideas for busy families.

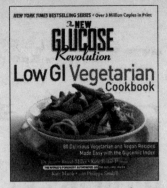

ISBN 978-1-56924-278-0 • $19.95

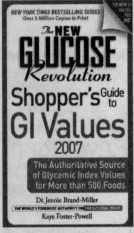

ISBN 978-1-56924-280-3 • $6.95

THE NEW GLUCOSE REVOLUTION SHOPPER'S GUIDE TO GI VALUES 2007

With GI values for hundreds of foods and beverages, this guide makes it easier than ever to ascertain a food's GI value. Included are: an A to Z listing that specifies serving size, net carbohydrate per serving, and the glycemic load, sorted according to low, intermediate, and high-GI values.

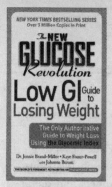

1-56924-336-7 • $6.95

THE NEW GLUCOSE REVOLUTION LOW GI GUIDE TO LOSING WEIGHT

Learn how you can best use the glycemic index for effective weight loss. *The New Glucose Revolution Low GI Guide to Losing Weight* clearly describes the differences between carbohydrates and how low-GI foods can help you feel fuller longer, burn more body fat, and achieve and maintain a healthy weight and life-long eating habits.

THE LOW GI DIET COOKBOOK

One hundred absolutely delicious, easy-to-make low-GI recipes—all of which feature low-GI carbohydrates—that will inspire you to adopt low-GI eating as *the* way to cook and eat—not only to keep your weight under control, but to improve and maintain your overall health and vitality, for life.

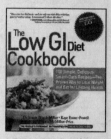

1-56924-359-X • $19.95

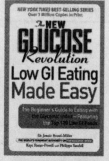

1-56924-385-9 • $12.95

THE NEW GLUCOSE REVOLUTION LOW GI EATING MADE EASY

A one-stop resource for those looking to switch to a healthy low-GI diet, this easy-to-follow guide features in-depth entries for the top 100 foods with the lowest GI values. Tips for making easy substitutions from high to low-GI foods and over 300 quick meal, snack, and treat suggestions are offered throughout.

Food manufacturers are showing increasing interest in having the GI values of their products measured. Some are already including the GI value of foods on food labels. As more and more research highlights the benefits of low-GI foods, consumers and dietitians are writing and telephoning food companies and diabetes organizations asking for GI data. This symbol has been registered in several countries, including the United States and Australia, to indicate that a food has been properly GI tested—in real people, not in a test tube—and also makes a positive contribution to nutrition. You can find out more about the program at www.gisymbol.com.au.

As consumers, you have a right to information about the nutrients and physiological effects of foods. You have a right to know the GI value of a food and to know it has been tested using appropriate standardized methodology.